POSITIONAL RELEASE THERAPY

Assessment & Treatment
of Musculoskeletal Dysfunction

POSITIONAL RELEASE THERAPY

Assessment & Treatment of Musculoskeletal Dysfunction

Kerry J. D'Ambrogio,
D.O.M., A.P., P.T., D.O.-M.T.P.

President, Therapeutic Systems, Inc.
Sarasota, Florida; www.TSItherapy.com
Faculty, Dialogues in Contemporary Rehabilitation
Hartford, Connecticut;
Faculty, Northeast Seminars
East Hampstead, New Hampshire;
Faculty, East West College of Natural Healing
Sarasota, Florida
Director of Manual Therapy, Upledger Institute
West Palm Beach, Florida

George B. Roth, B.Sc., D.C., N.D.

Faculty, Department of Post-graduate and
 Continuing Education
Canadian Memorial Chiropractic College;
Director, Wellness Institute
Toronto, Canada;
President, Wellness Systems, Inc.
Caledon, Canada;
Industrial Injury Prevention Consultant

with illustrations by
Jeanne Robertson

with photographs by
Stuart Halperin
and Matthew Wiley

with 256 illustrations
with 342 photographs

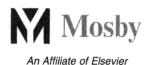

An Affiliate of Elsevier

An Affiliate of Elsevier

Vice President and Publisher: Don Ladig
Executive Editor: Martha Sasser
Associate Developmental Editor: Amy Dubin
Developmental Editor: Kellie White
Project Manager: Dana Peick
Project Specialist: Catherine Albright
Designer: Amy Buxton
Manufacturing Manager: Betty Richmond
Cover Art: Leonardo Da Vinci

Permissions may be sought directly from Elsevier's Science and Technology Rights Department in
Oxford, UK. Phone: (44) 1865 843830, Fax: (44) 1865 853333, e-mail: permissions@elsevier.co.uk.
You may also complete your request on-line via the Elsevier homepage: http://www.elsevier.com by
selecting "Customer Support" and then "Obtaining Permissions".

ISBN-13: 978-0-8151-0096-6
ISBN-10:   0-8151-0096-5

Mosby
11830 Westline Industrial Drive
St. Louis, Missouri 63146

Library of Congress Cataloging-in-Publication Data

D'Ambrogio, Kerry J.
    Positional release therapy: assessment and treatment of
musculoskeletal dysfunction / Kerry J. D'Ambrogio, George B. Roth ;
with illustrations by Jeanne Robertson.
        p.   cm.
    Includes bibliographical references and index.
    ISBN-13: 978-0-8151-0096-6   ISBN-10: 0-8151-0096-5
    1. Manipulation (Therapeutics)   2. Soft tissue injuries.
3. Musculoskeletal system—Wounds and injuries.   I. Roth, George B.
II. Title
    [DNLM: 1. Manipulation, Orthopedic—methods.   2. Pain—therapy.
3. Soft Tissue Injuries—therapy.   WB 535 D156p 1997]
    RZ341.D18 1997
    616.7'062—dc20
    DNLM/DLC
                                                                        96-25538

About the Authors

KERRY J. D'AMBROGIO, D.O.M., A.P., P.T., D.O.-M.T.P.
Dr. Kerry D'Ambrogio, D.O.M., A.P., P.T., D.O.-M.T.P., is a Board Certified Acupuncture Physician, Physical Therapist, and Osteopath (Canada). Kerry graduated from the University of Toronto, Canada in Physical Therapy, the Academy of Chinese Healing Arts in Acupuncture and the Canadian Academy of Osteopathy and Health Sciences in Osteopathy. He has studied a great number of manual therapy and exercise courses from around the world in the Osteopathic, Chiropractic, and Physical Therapy professions. This diverse background provides Kerry with an integrated approach in the evaluation and treatment of musculoskeletal dysfunction and rehabilitation. Kerry has been actively involved in teaching seminars and speaking at research, physical therapy, chiropractic and athletic therapy conventions throughout Canada, the United States, Mexico, South America, Europe, Middle East, Africa, China, Japan, Australia and New Zealand. He is the founder of Therapeutic System, Incorporated (T.S.I.), an international seminar company. He is a certified instructor recognized by the International Alliance of Healthcare Educators (IAHE). Kerry was the Director of the Manual Therapy Curriculum at the Upledger Institute, and was on faculty with Dialogues in Contemporary Rehabilitation (D.C.R.), Northeast Seminars and East West College of Natural Medicine. Kerry has contributed a chapter in a published manual therapy textbook and has been interviewed on radio to educate the public regarding manual therapy. Kerry currently lives in Bradenton, Florida with his wife Jane and three children, Carli, Cassi, and Blake. His practice is at 7311 Merchant Court, Sarasota, Florida 34240.
Phone: 941.907.9250. **Email:** TSIseminar@aol.com **Web site:** www.TSItherapy.com

GEORGE B. ROTH, B.Sc., D.C., N.D.
Dr. George Roth holds a Bachelor of Science degree from the University of Toronto and doctorates in Chiropractic and Naturopathic Medicine. He has been internationally recognized in the field of musculoskeletal therapy and invited to present at many physical medicine, chiropractic and athletic injury conferences. He has conducted seminars at the post-graduate level co-sponsored by Logan College of Chiropractic in St. Louis, Missouri, the Canadian Memorial Chiropractic College in Toronto and Physical Medicine Research Foundation. He has also presented seminars to the University of Western Ontario, Dept. of Physiotherapy/Athletic Injuries; the American Back Society; the University of Toronto Faculty of Medicine, and at numerous hospital and university based symposia throughout North America. He has also appeared on radio and television to discuss a variety of health-related topics and has been retained to treat the cast and crew in movies and television productions. Dr. Roth is in private practice and is also on staff at a large sports injury clinic, treating professional and Olympic athletes. He has also developed a revolutionary rehabilitation program for racehorses. He is an experienced clinician, who has made it his life's work to investigate the underlying mechanisms behind health and disease and, through the Roth Institute, continues to research, practice, teach and write on these subjects.

Dedication

The authors would like to dedicate this book to Dr. Lawrence Jones, D.O., F.A.A.O. (1912-1996) for his pioneering discoveries in the field of musculoskeletal treatment and his contributions to the service of mankind. Dr. Jones spent over 40 years developing Strain-Counterstrain. During the process he gave his time, energy, and talent so that future generations of practitioners could enhance the care of their patients. His contributions have gained the respect and admiration of a broad spectrum of health professionals worldwide. Dr. Jones made it his life's work to share his knowledge for the benefit of others. We hope that our contribution to this continuing work will do his memory justice.

Forewords

The body is a symphony of movement orchestrated by the natural oscillations of its component parts. The beat starts at the cellular (probably subcellular) level with the oscillations of the individual cells. The organs, the heart, the lungs, the brain and spinal fluid, the gut, kidneys, liver, and muscles all contribute their rhythm, pitch, and timbre, first to their organ system, and then to the orchestrated body. When it all functions together, it is a harmonic work of great complexity. When one of the players misses a beat it can produce a discordant mess. The New York Academy of Sciences has held conferences on the nature of biologic rhythms and their dysfunctions and uses the terms *dynamic diseases* to describe the illnesses caused by these arrythmias. These are disorders of systems that can be described as a breakdown of the control or coordinating mechanisms, in which systems that normally oscillate stop oscillating or begin to oscillate in new and unexpected ways.

To many of us in the field of musculoskeletal medicine it has become apparent that what we treat is usually not pathology in the classic Vercovian model, where each disease has a verifiable tissue injury or biochemical disorder, but rather a perturbation of the normal rhythms of the musculoskeletal system—a dynamic disease. New models that can explain both the static and dynamic mechanical functions of the body as an integrated whole are being developed. In these models the body is a nonlinear, hierarchical, structural system with every part functioning independently and as part of the whole, like instruments in a symphony orchestra. How do we fix what is out of tune?

Dynamic systems function nonlinearly. Linear processes, once out of whack, tend to stay out of whack. Nonlinear processes tend to be self-correcting. A slight nudge may encourage a nonlinear process to correct itself. We take advantage of this when we jar a dysfunctional television set, scare away a hiccup, or defibrillate a heart. In the musculoskeletal system practitioners may treat similar problems with a variety of interventions. Joint manipulation of various ilk, cranial manipulation, acupuncture, massage, exercise, and so on all seem to work, in the right hands and at the right time, often for the same problem. John Mennell, a pioneer in the field of musculoskeletal medicine, said that if practitioner A is using method A to treat a perceived problem and practitioner B is using method B to treat the same problem as he or she perceives it, and they are both successful in their outcome, then they must both be doing the same thing to the same thing, no matter what they say they are seeing or doing. I suspect that we are all treating mechanical discords of the musculoskeletal system, interferences with the normal oscillations that we, somehow, may set right.

George Roth and Kerry D'Ambrogio have put all these thoughts together in an insightful book. They recognize the oneness of the musculoskeletal system and have built on the work of others to devise a treatment method based on scientific principles of nonlinear dynamic systems. If there is a musculoskeletal dysfunction, we may be able to facilitate the normal rhythms of the system by stopping the orchestra, giving it a downbeat, and allowing the natural oscillations, built into the structure, to get things back in tune. This is the principle used in defibrillating a dysfunctional heart by shocking it still, and it seems to be the principle underlying positional release therapy.

Positional release therapy is remarkably simple and is guided by the recognized diagnostic duo of somatic dysfunction (which is characterized as loss of joint play at the joint level and similar tissue restrictions at each level studied) and tender points (which are unrelated to local inflammation or injury). These appear to be the diagnostic sine qua non of dynamic diseases of the musculoskeletal system. Learning is made easy by this copiously illustrated book that is both a "how to" manual and a "why for" text. The marriage of the two disciplines, chiropractic and physical therapy, makes this a particularly important book. However, as pointed out by George and Kerry, this is a book for all practitioners in the field of musculoskeletal medicine. Because the technique is so simple, safe, and easy to learn, it can serve as an introduction to musculoskeletal techniques for the less skilled and also as a valuable adjunct technique for the more experienced practitioner. It is a powerful tool that should be included in every clinician's bag.

Stephen M. Levin, M.D., F.A.C.S.
Director, Potomac Back Center
Vienna, Virginia

Positional release therapy is an extraordinary means of reducing hypertonicity, both protective muscle spasm and the spasticity of neurologic manifestation. Its great achievements are correction of joint hypomobility, improvement of articular balance (which is the normal relationship between two articular surfaces throughout a full range of physiologic motion), elongation of the muscle fiber during relaxation, and increase in soft tissue flexibility secondary to reduced excessive sensory input into the central nervous system. Pain and disability may be remarkably reduced with this approach.

Therapists and physicians can use *Positional Release Therapy: Assessment and Treatment of Musculoskeletal Dysfunction* with almost every patient, in all fields of health care. Orthopedic patients enjoy improved function and decreased pain with increased motion. Chronic pain patients experience decreased discomfort, possibly less inflammation, and more functional movement. Neurologic patients, when this approach is slightly adapted to meet their unique requirements, attain positive gains in tone reduction with improved function in all aspects of activities of daily living. Positional release therapy is a comprehensive approach for all persons with stress-induced and dysfunction-induced muscle fiber contraction.

Dr. Lawrence Jones introduced the correction of musculoskeletal dysfunction by correlating tender points with positions of comfort as described in his book *Strain and Counterstrain*. He based his findings on the theory that the treatment positions resulted in a reduction of neuronal activity within the myotatic reflex arc. Kerry D'Ambrogio and George Roth have extended and organized this approach and have included several new theories to account for the clinical manifestations. They have provided a total body scanning process for increased efficiency in practice management. Muscle and tissue references are listed, to provide a clear and pertinent anatomic and kinesiologic basis for treatment. The photographs and illustrations are remarkably supportive for the study and practice of these techniques. Body mechanics, as it relates to the reduction of strain on the patient and the practitioner, are addressed in some detail.

Positional Release Therapy: Assessment and Treatment of Musculoskeletal Dysfunction is an exceptional textbook that addresses neuromusculoskeletal dysfunction in an effective and efficient manner. My belief is that their work will enhance our goal of improving health care through the use of manual therapy.

My personal thanks are extended to Dr. Lawrence Jones for his landmark contribution of strain and counterstrain technique. My patients will be forever grateful. And my congratulations are extended to George Roth and Kerry D'Ambrogio for this valuable new book.

Sharon Weiselfish, Ph.D., P.T.
Co-partner, Regional Physical Therapy
West Hartford, Plainville, and South Windsor, Connecticut
Co-partner, Mobile Therapy Associates
Glastonbury, Connecticut;
Director, Dialogues in Contemporary Research (D.C.R.)
Hartford, Connecticut

Acknowledgments

Many people over the years have helped to develop my belief system with regard to my healing and treatment intervention philosophies. It is sometimes difficult to say where specific ideas originated because all these people shared similar beliefs. I would like to acknowledge this outstanding group of professionals for helping me put this book together. It has been an honor to be associated with those who are so dedicated to sharing their knowledge, thoughts, and ideas over the years:

John Barnes, P.T., Jean Pierre Barral, D.O., Paul Chauffeur, D.O., Doug Freer, P.T., Dr. Dan Gleason, D.C., Phillip Greenman, D.O., Dr. Vladmir Janda, M.D., P.T., Dr. Lawrence Jones, D.O., Dr. David Leaf, D.C., Goldie Lewis, P.T., Frank Lowen, L.M.T., Edward Stiles, D.O., Dr. Fritz Smith, D.O., John Upledger, D.O., Dr. Todd Bezilla, D.O., Robert Johnston, D.O.-M.T.P. Andrew Puchta, D.O.-M.T.P, Brandon Stevens, D.O.-M.T.P. And Sharon Weiselfish, Ph.D., P.T. Thanks again to Doug Freer who originally inspired me.

Thanks to Jane D'Ambrogio, B.A., B.Ed., Conrad Penner, P.T., and Sharon Weiselfish, PH.D., P.T., for editing chapters and for constructive advice and support.

I would like to thank Dr. George Roth, D.C., for his patience and guidance. I've enjoyed the collaboration, friendship, and learning experiences in the writing of this book.

A special thanks to Sharon Weiselfish, Ph.D., P.T. for her friendship, contributions, insight, and support.

Most of all, I'd like thank my loving wife Jane, my kids Carli, Cassi, and Blake, and my Mom and Dad, who have provided me with the love and support needed to write this book. They have contended with more than anyone with regard to time spent and patience required, in writing this book.

Sincere thanks to all of you.
Kerry J. D'Ambrogio D.O.M., A.P., P.T., D.O.-M.T.P

I would like to thank Harold Schwartz, D.O., for helping to resolve my back pain and for opening me up to a new way of looking at the body. Dr. Lawrence Jones inspired me through his down-to-earth common sense and his humility, and I hope that he would find this book a worthy testament to his goal of bringing these therapies to the world.

Several gifted practitioners, whom I can also call friends, have been a continuing source of constructive criticism as positional release therapy has evolved over the years: Garry Lapenskie, P.T., Stephen Levin, M.D., F.A.C.S., Iris Weverman, P.T., Iris Marshall, M.D., Heather Hartsell, Ph.D., P.T., and Cecil Eaves, R.M.T., Ph.D. I am specifically grateful to Garry Lapenskie, P.T., for his help in editing the manuscript. Stephen Levin, M.D., has been a continuing source of inspiration and a good friend.

Working with Kerry has been stimulating, and I feel that, despite occasional challenges, we have become better friends and developed a greater respect for each other through this collaboration. It can truly be said that the whole is greater than the sum of each of our parts.

Last, but not least, I wish to thank my loving wife Deborah and my son Joshua for their love and support. The past 2 years has been a strain on them because of the long hours I spent on this book, often hibernating away well into the night with my computer to write and edit the text. I cannot begin to express my gratitude for their patience with their part-time husband and dad during this time.

George B. Roth

Kerry and George would both like to thank the following:

Photographers Stuart Halperin and Matthew Wiley and illustrator Jeanne Robertson for their professionalism, patience, and remarkable talents. They have created an incredible visual learning experience for the reader.

Models Mary-Ellen McKenna, N.D., Carol Fisher-Short, R.M.T., and Robin Whale, D.C., for the long hours they put in and an extra thanks to Robin and Mary-Ellen for the second photo shoot.

Mosby staff Amy Dubin, Kellie White, Catherine Albright, and Martha Sasser for their advice, support, and patience with timelines.

Preface

"The magic is not in the medicine but in the patient's body - in the vis medicatrix naturae, the recuperative or self-corrective energy of nature. What the treatment does is to stimulate natural functions or to remove what hinders them."

Miracles, C.S. Lewis, 1940

The purpose of this book is to provide the practitioner with a powerful set of tools to precisely and consistently resolve difficult cases of soft tissue injury and musculoskeletal dysfunction. This text is an attempt to bring this information to the reader in a format that is concise, orderly, and user-friendly. We have formulated a system of assessment and treatment that can be easily learned and readily used to benefit patients. This material is appropriate for physical therapists, chiropractors, osteopaths, medical practitioners, occupational therapists, athletic trainers, and massage therapists.

We acknowledge the pioneers in this field for their contributions and view this text as a step toward a greater understanding of the complex nature of the human body. We are hopeful that this work will represent a measure of progress in the field of musculoskeletal therapy and enhance the clinical applicability of these powerful techniques.

The basis of the treatment program described in this text can be traced to related practices in antiquity. In this century, positional release therapy (PRT) has evolved through the work of various clinicians, but the discovery of the clinical application of these principles is credited primarily to Dr. Lawrence H. Jones, D.O. His dedication to uncovering the basic principles of this form of therapy was a monumental achievement. Jones exemplifies the essence of Thomas Edison's definition: "Intelligence is perseverance in disguise." He is recognized as one of the great pioneers in the field of musculoskeletal therapy.

Positional release therapy has had a powerful impact on both of us in terms of clinical success and patient acceptance. In addition, our personal experience in dealing with our own painful conditions was instrumental in directing us to the development of this art.

In George's case a severe, chronic condition of upper back pain developed subsequent to a motor vehicle acci-

dent that occured during childhood. The condition was exacerbated periodically on exertion. After becoming a chiropractor, George began seeking more effective and gentle methods of treatment, which eventually led him to study with several prominent osteopaths. He read an article by Jones that described counterstrain and subsequently met Dr. Harold Schwartz, D.O. (a student of Jones), who was the head of the department of osteopathic medicine at a prominent teaching hospital. At about this time, George was experiencing an acute episode of his back condition that prevented him from sleeping in a recumbent position. It had proved resistant to several other modalities over the previous 3 months and was relieved by Schwartz in less than 10 minutes.

This experience motivated him to begin a concerted quest to uncover the mysteries of this amazing therapy. He spent the next 5 years commuting between Toronto and Columbus in order to continue studying with Schwartz and eventually with Jones. George then began assisting and coteaching with Jones and developed courses for chiropractors, physical therapists, and other practitioners throughout Canada. He also developed a specialized treatment table that was designed to facilitate the application of this form of therapy.

While playing varsity football at the University of Western Ontario, Kerry D'Ambrogio experienced several recurring injuries to his groin, hip flexors, and right knee. These injuries plagued him during his 3 years at Western and limited his activity. As a result, he spent some time in the athletic injury clinic and received traditional therapy, which consisted of cold whirlpools, ultrasound, and stretching. While attending therapy Kerry observed other athletes being treated, and this exposure sparked an interest in physical therapy. He decided to enter into studies at the University of Toronto to become a physical therapist. Throughout this period he continued to suffer from chronic pain.

Kerry was first exposed to counterstrain by his professor, Doug Freer, and eventually attended a workship with Jones. At the workship, Kerry discovered several severe tender points in his pelvic region and one on his right patellar tendon. Upon treatment, he experienced a dramatic improvement in the function of his pelvis, hip, and right knee. Consequently, he was able to fully resume sports activities. This one treatment was able to accomplish more than the countless previous therapy sessions. This extraordinary response motivated Kerry to pursue the study of counterstrain. He eventually assisted with Jones and then developed his own series of seminars so that he could share this technique with other professionals.

Both of us had been exploring soft tissue skills over the past several years and found that our paths were intersecting along synchronous lines as we pursued this knowledge. We both became involved with teaching and writing manuals for our seminars. When the idea to write a formal text was presented to George, he contacted Kerry, who, suprisingly, had been thinking of writing a book as well. The collaboration naturally evolved and was seen by both of us as a unique opportunity to provide a greater degree of depth to the material and intergrate the concepts of chiropractic, osteopathy, and physical therapy.

We have attempted to provide a theoretical and historical perspective for positional release therapy. This foundation is intended to support the clinical experience and provide a level of confidence in the rationale for these techniques. An awareness and understanding of the underlying principles and context of a therapeutic model can play an important role in sustaining the perseverance required to develop the skills necessary for its application.

The reader is provided with criteria for deciding whether it is appropriate to utilize PRT as a treatment modality. With the numerous emerging therapies available to the student of musculoskeletal therapy, we felt that is was necessary to provide a "road map" in order to plot a course of appropriate treatment. It should be noted that PRT is *not* a panacea and is best utilized within a complementary range of therapeutic options as indicated for each individual patient.

An outline of general treatment principles and rules is presented to provide a framework for consistent application of the procedures. These guidelines have been established during the past 30 to 40 years and can serve to increase efficiency and save the therapist from repeating much of the trial and error that was involved in the evolution of this approach. The clinician is also encouraged to perform a number of *reality checks* to establish clinical indexes for improved function. These can include standard orthopedic and neurologic tests and specialized functional procedures. (See Chapter 7.)

The *scanning evaluation* (SE), discussed in Chapter 5, and provided in its entirety in the Appendix, is designed to facilitate the cataloguing of the tender points. The SE provides a system to organize assessment findings and serves as a reference that quickly allows the practitioner to determine a prioritized treatment program. This format can save a great deal of time and provides an efficient method to track progress of the patient's condition and plan subsequent treatments.

Jones coined the terms *counterstrain* and *strain and counterstrain* (the latter being the title of his orginal text). Several authors, including Jones, have referred to the general therapeutic approach as release by positioning and positional release therapy. We feel that the term *positional release therapy* best describes this form of therapy in its broader, generic sense.

With respect to the terminology used in the treatment section, we have endeavored to keep this as simple as possible while attempting to maintain a degree of structural relevance. In certain cases, the terminology as coined by Jones is used; however, every attempt was made to correlate the treatment approach to the anatomic tissues involved. In a few instances, a positional reference is used where this has been determined to be the most logical format. Abbreviations have been assigned for each treatment; these consist of two to four letters plus numeral designations. For those trained in the Jones method, a cross-reference with PRT terminology is provided (see the Appendix). There is also a cross-reference in the Appendix that correlates muscles and other tissues with the appropriate PRT treatment. This can be used to quickly locate a particular treatment according to the involved tissue.

Modifications of treatment positions and changes in terminology are intended to improve the efficiency of treatment and simplify the recording and communication of clinical findings. These changes should not detract from previous discoveries but will hopefully serve to continue the development of this art and science. Evolution is a process of building on previously established foundations.

The description of the point locations and treatment procedures represents the core of this text. The underlying principle in the design of the illustrations and photographs has been to clearly portray the location of the tender points, the anatomic structures involved, and the general position of treatment. The treatment section is divided into upper quadrant and lower quadrant sections. Each region of the body (cranium, cervical spine, thoracic spine, upper limb, etc.) is prefaced by an introduction to its clinical relevance and general guidelines for the application of PRT. Each region is also headed by anatomic illustrations outlining the general location of the most common tender points. Each tender point or group of tender points has a separate page that consists of a photograph and illustration with the specific point location, detailed photographs of the treatment positions, and written descriptions of the location of the tender points and the position of treatment.

Chapter 7 provides a realistic clinical context to the application of PRT. Strategies to help refine the techniques and optimize results are provided, as well as modifications for dealing with special clinical challenges. This chapter addresses the subtleties of the *art* of application of PRT skills. Potential pitfalls and questions related to clinical issues are also addressed.

We hope that this text will inspire the reader to look at musculoskeletal disorders in new ways. The inherent, self-healing potential of the body deserves our respect and support in the spirit of *primum no nocere* (first do no harm). We believe that positional release therapy is an approach that embraces this ideal and is truly powerful in its gentleness. We are hopeful that this work will be of value to you, the practitioner. The relief of pain and the improved function of your patients will be the ultimate measure of our success.

Contents

Positional Release Therapy

Assessment & Treatment of Musculoskeletal Dysfunction

1

Origins of Positional Release Therapy

The purpose of this chapter is to trace the development of positional release therapy (PRT) and put it into historical perspective. Positional release therapy is an indirect technique; it places the body into a position of greatest comfort and employs tender points to identify and monitor the lesion. Because PRT appears to be an effective modality, it must be based on certain general principles that have a sound physiologic basis. Several of the characteristics of PRT, which may be shared with other therapeutic models, can be identified. These include the use of *body positioning*, the use of *tender points* to identify the lesion and to monitor the therapeutic intervention, and an *indirect* approach with respect to tissue resistance.

¶BODY POSITIONING

Body posture and the relative position of body parts has been a subject of intense speculation and research throughout history. From yoga to the martial arts to the study of body language, the arrangement of the parts of the human body has been deemed to have a certain mental, physical, and spiritual significance. Several forms of yoga, a discipline with over 5000 years of history, include the physical practice of positioning the body to enhance function and release tension.[17] These positions put certain parts of the body under stretch while other parts are placed in a position of relaxation (Fig. 1-1). The benefits of this form of exercise to relieve musculoskeletal pain are widely accepted, and they are used successfully by a substantial number of people.[10,22] Modern derivations of this ancient art may be seen in the practices of Feldenkrais, bioenergetic

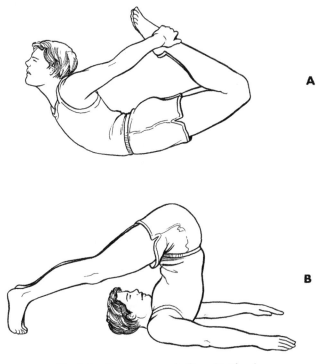

Fig. 1-1 *Yoga postures.* **A**, *Bow.* **B**, *Plough.*

therapy, sotai, core stabilization, functional technic, and counterstrain (Fig. 1-2).* These practices share a commonality in that they recognize the relationship of body movement and posture with the general condition of the body.

---

*References 1,7,9,10,11,15,17.

1

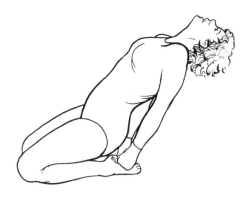

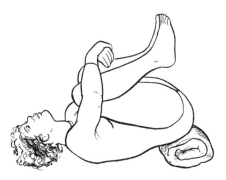

Fig. 1-2 *Bioenergetic exercises.* (Modified from Lowen A, Lowen L: *The way to vibrant health: a manual of bioenergetic exercises,* New York, 1974, Harper & Row.)

Several authors, both modern and ancient, elaborate on the "energetic" properties of postures and body positions.[30,31,35] Some of these phenomena have been noted regularly by practitioners of PRT as part of the release process, which is discussed in later chapters. The mechanism responsible for these effects is unknown.

¶TENDER POINTS

Acupuncture points have been used therapeutically for at least 5000 years. These points correlate closely with many of those "discovered" by subsequent investigators (Fig. 1-3).[36] References in the western literature to the presence of palpable tender points (TPs) within muscle date back to 1843. Froriep described his so-called Muskelschwiele, or muscle callus, which referred to the tender points in muscle that were found to be associated with rheumatic conditions. In 1876 the Swedish investigator Helleday described tender points and nodules in cases of chronic myositis. In 1904 Gowers introduced the term *fibrositis* to describe the palpable nodule, which he felt was associated with the fibrous elements of the musculoskeletal system. Postmortem studies by Schade, which were reported in Germany in 1919, demonstrated thickened nodules in muscle, which served to confirm that these histologic changes evolved into lesions that were independent of ongoing proximal neurologic excitation.[33] In the 1930s Chapman[5] discovered a system of

reflexes that he associated with the functioning of the lymphatic system (Fig. 1-4). He found that direct treatment of these reflex tender areas resulted in improved circulation and lymphatic drainage. Resolution of the underlying condition, whether visceral or musculoskeletal, reduced the tenderness of these areas. These reflexes have been described as gangliform contractions within the deep fascia that are about the size of a pea. More recently, Travell and Simons[33] have systematized the mapping and direct treatment of TPs in their two-volume series, *Myofascial Pain and Dysfunction.* Jones[14] reported on his discovery of tender points associated with musculoskeletal dysfunction as early as 1964. The recognition of the tender point, or trigger point, as an important pathophysiologic indicator of musculoskeletal dysfunction has also been elaborated by Rosomoff.[23,24]

Bosey[2] states that acupuncture points are situated in palpable depressions—*cupules*—under which lie fibrous cones containing neurovascular formations associated with concentrations of free nerve endings, Golgi endings, and Pacini corpuscles. Melzack and associates[19] contend that there are no major differences between tender points, trigger points, acupuncture points, or other reflex tender areas that have been described by different investigators. The varying effects reported with the use of different tender points may lie in their relative location with respect to underlying tissues. Chaitow[3] points out that so-called spontaneous sensitive points arise as the result of trauma or musculoskeletal dysfunction. The Chinese refer to these points as Ah Shi points in their writings dating back to the Tang dynasty (618–907 AD). Chaitow[4] insists that these are identical to the points used by Jones.

In summary, tender points have been recognized for thousands of years as having diagnostic and therapeutic significance. Various investigators have rediscovered these points and have applied a range of therapeutic interventions to influence them. In general, any therapy that is able to reduce the tenderness of these tissues appears to have a beneficial effect on the health of the individual. Jones[14] was the first clinician to associate body position with a reduction in sensitivity of these tender points.

¶INDIRECT TECHNIQUE

The history of therapeutic intervention to affect somatic structures can be broadly divided into *direct* and *indirect* techniques. Direct techniques involve force being applied against a resistance barrier, such as stretching, joint mobilization, and muscle energy.[8,20] Indirect techniques employ the application of force away from a resistance barrier, that is, in the direction of greatest ease. Indirect therapies, including PRT, have evolved in various forms and share certain common characteristics and underlying principles.

In 1943 Sutherland[32] introduced the concept of manipulation of cranial structures. His technique to treat cra-

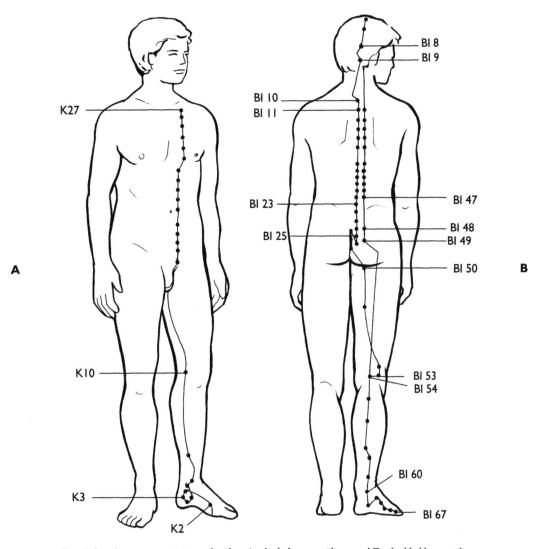

Fig. 1-3 *Acupuncture points related to* **A,** *the kidney meridian; and* **B,** *the bladder meridian.*

nial lesions was to follow the motion of the skull in the direction in which it moved most freely. By placing pressure on the bones of the head in the direction of greatest ease, he found that the tissues spontaneously relaxed and allowed for a normalization of structural alignment and function.

In the late 1940s Hoover[11] introduced *functional technic.* He found that when a body part or joint was placed in a position of *dynamic reciprocal balance,* in which all tensions were equal, the body would spontaneously release the restrictions associated with the lesion. During that period, the prevailing view of musculoskeletal assessment stressed the position and morphology of body parts. Hoover emphasized the importance of "listening" to the tissues, which refers to the process of carefully observing, through palpation, the patterns of tension within the tissues and paying attention to their functional characteristics and structure. He introduced the concept of *functional diagnosis,* which takes into account the range of motion and tissue play within the structures being assessed.

Hoover advocated a treatment protocol that was respectful of the wisdom of the tissues and the inherent interaction of the neuromuscular, myofascial, and articular components. The technique involves movement toward least resistance and greatest comfort and relies on the response of tissues under the palpating hand of the practitioner. This *dynamic neutral* position attempts to reproduce a balance of tensions, which is near the anatomic neutral position for the joint, within its traumatically induced range. A series of tissue changes may occur during the positioning that are perceived by the practitioner. The practitioner attempts to follow this evolving pattern until the body spontaneously achieves a state of resolution and treatment is complete.[11]

Jones[15] found that specific positions were able to reduce the sensitivity of tender points. Once located, the tender point is maintained with the palpating finger at a subthreshold pressure. The patient is then passively placed in a position that reduces the tension under the palpating finger and causes a subjective reduction in tenderness as reported by

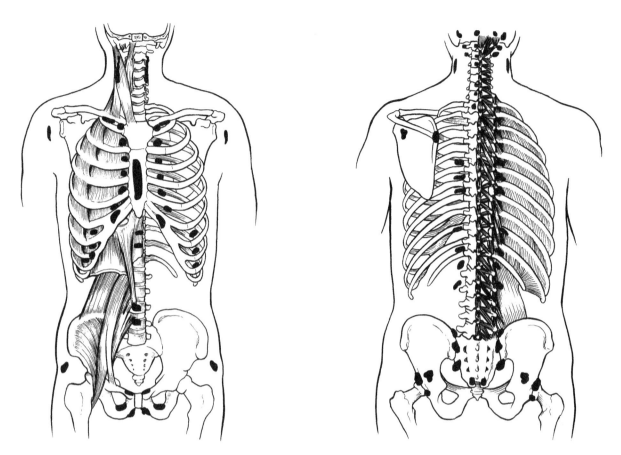

Fig. 1-4   *Chapman's reflexes.* (Modified from Chaitow L: *Soft tissue manipulation,* Rochester, Vt, 1988, Healing Arts Press.)

the patient.[15] This "specific" position is, nevertheless, fine-tuned throughout the treatment period (90 seconds), much in the way that Hoover follows the lesion in his technique. Chaitow[4] also alludes to the possibility that a therapeutic effect is exerted by maintaining contact with the tender point.

In 1963 Rumney[27] described the basis for reestablishing normal spinal motion as "inherent corrective forces of the body—if the patient is properly positioned, his own natural forces may restore normal motion to an area." Other clinicians have used an indirect method to treat musculoskeletal dysfunction by having patients actively position themselves through various ranges of motion under the guidance of the practitioner and while being monitored for maximal ease by palpation.[8,18]

¶HISTORY OF COUNTERSTRAIN

In 1954 Lawrence H. Jones, an osteopath with almost 20 years of experience, was called on by a patient who had been suffering with low back pain of 2 months' duration that had not responded to chiropractic care. The patient displayed an apparent psoas spasm with resultant antalgic posture. Jones was determined that he could succeed where others had failed. However, after several sessions with no improvement, he was ready to admit defeat in the face of this resistant case. The patient was in so much pain that

sleep for more than a few minutes was impossible. Jones decided that finding a comfortable position that would allow the patient to sleep would at least provide some temporary relief and some much-needed rest. After much trial and error, they found a comfortable position. Jones propped the patient in this unusual-looking folded position with several pillows and left him to rest. Upon his return some time later, Jones suggested that the patient memorize the position in order to reproduce it when going to bed that night. The patient was then slowly taken out of the position and instructed to stand up. Much to the amazement of the patient and Jones, the patient stood erect and with drastically reduced pain. In the words of Jones, "the patient was delighted and I was dumbfounded!"[14,15]

This discovery emphasized the value of the position of comfort. Jones found that by maintaining these positions for varying periods of time, lasting improvement would often be the result. He initially held the position for 20 minutes and gradually found that 90 seconds was the minimal threshold for optimal correction of the lesion.

As Jones pursued the possible applications of this new discovery, which he referred to as counterstrain, he noted that many of the painful conditions that he was able to alleviate were associated with the presence of acutely painful tender points. The traditional approach to lesions of the spine was to assess and treat on the basis of tender areas in the paraspinal tissues. These points, after positioning of the patient, became decidedly reduced in tenderness and remained so even after the treatment was concluded. Thus an important diagnostic dimension was added to this form of therapy.

In many instances of back and neck pain, however, no tender point could be found in the area of the pain within the paraspinal tissues. Fate was once again to play a role. A patient who had been seeing Jones for low back pain was working in the garden when he was struck in the groin with a rake handle. In pain and fearing that he may have induced a hernia, he called on Jones. Jones examined the patient and assured him that no hernia was present. Jones then decided that the patient might as well stay and receive a treatment that was scheduled for later in the week. After the patient had been placed in the position for treatment of his low back, in which he was supine and flexed maximally at the hips, Jones decided to recheck the previously tender area in the groin. To his surprise, the tenderness was gone. This discovery answered the mystery of the missing tender points, and shortly thereafter Jones was able to uncover an array of anteriorly located tender points that were associated with pain throughout the spine.[13] He noted that approximately 30% to 50% of back pain was associated with these anterior tender points. With this latter discovery, much of the guesswork and trial and error in the application of therapy was eliminated. The use of tender points became a reliable indicator of the type of lesion being encountered, and therapeutic intervention could thus be instituted with increased confidence and reproducibility. Jones spent the better part of 30 years developing and documenting his discoveries, which he first published in 1964.[14] He later produced a book entitled *Strain and Counterstrain*.[15]

¶ RECENT ADVANCES

Positional release therapy owes its recent evolution to a number of clinicians and researchers. Schwartz[29] adapted several techniques to reduce practitioner strain. Shiowitz[28] introduced the use of a facilitating force (compression, torsion, etc.) to enhance the effect of the positioning. Ramirez and others[21] discovered a group of tender points on the posterior aspect of the sacrum that have significant connections to the pelvic mechanism. Weiselfish[34] outlined the specific application of positional release techniques for use with the neurologic patient. She found that the initial phase of release (neuromuscular) required a minimum of 3 minutes, and she also outlined protocols to locate key areas of involvement with this patient population. She, along with one of us (D'Ambrogio), outlined the two phases of release: neuromuscular and myofascial. Brown[1] developed a system of exercise for the spine in which a pain-free range of motion is maintained. One of us (D'Ambrogio) developed the *scanning evaluation* procedure to facilitate the efficiency and thoroughness of patient assessment,[6] and one of us (Roth) has developed improved practitioner body mechanics to reduce strain and has correlated lesions with

specific anatomic structures.[25] We have helped simplify the terminology used to describe lesions and systematized the educational program to help make the development of PRT skills more efficient. In the next chapter we will help to establish a physiologic basis for many of the clinical manifestations of musculoskeletal dysfunction.

¶ SUMMARY

Positional release therapy has historical roots in antiquity. The three major characteristics (body positioning, the use of tender points, and the indirect nature of the therapy) can be individually traced to practices established over the past 5000 years. Connections can be made with the ancient disciplines of yoga and acupuncture and with the work of investigators over the course of the past two centuries. The correlation of different systems that use tender points suggests a common mechanism for the development of these lesions. Significant contributions to the development of this art and science have been made by Jones[12,13,16] and others. Positional release therapy is being continually advanced and developed through the contributions of many clinicians and researchers.

References

1. Brown CW: Change in disc treatment saves hockey star, *Backletter* 7(12):1, 1992.
2. Bosey J: The morphology of acupuncture points, *Acupunc Electother Res* 2:79, 1984.
3. Chaitow L: *Soft tissue manipulation*, Rochester, Vt, 1988, Healing Arts Press.
4. Chaitow L: *The acupuncture treatment of pain*, Wellingborough, 1976, Thorsons.
5. Chapman F, Owens C: *Introduction to and endocrine interpretation of Chapman's reflexes*, self-published.
6. D'Ambrogio K: *Strain/counterstrain* (course syllabus), Palm Beach Gardens, 1992, Upledger Institute.
7. Feldenkrais M: *Awareness through movement: health exercises for personal growth*, New York, 1972, Harper & Row.
8. Greenman PE: *Principles of manual medicine*, Baltimore, 1989, Williams & Wilkins.
9. Hashimoto K: *Sotai natural exercise*, Oroville, Calif, 1981, George Ohsawa Macrobiotic Foundation.
10. Hewitt J: *The complete yoga book*, New York, 1977, Random House.
11. Hoover HV: Functional technic, *AAO Year Book* 47, 1958.
12. Jones LH: Foot treatment without hand trauma, *J Am Osteopath Assoc* 72:481, 1973.
13. Jones LH: Missed anterior spinal lesions: a preliminary report, *DO* 6:75, 1966.
14. Jones LH: Spontaneous release by positioning, *DO* 4:109, 1964.
15. Jones LH: *Strain and counterstrain*, Newark, Ohio, 1981, American Academy of Osteopathy.
16. Jones LH: Strain and counterstrain lectures at Jones Institute, 1992-1993.
17. Lowen A, Lowen L: *The way to vibrant health: a manual of bioenergetic exercises*, New York, 1974, Harper & Row.
18. Maigue R: The concept of painlessness and opposite motion in spinal manipulations, *Am J Phys Med* 44:55, 1965.
19. Melzack R, Stillwell DM, Fex EJ: Trigger points and acupuncture points for pain: correlations and implications, *Pain* 3:3, 1977.
20. Mitchell FL, Moran PS, Pruzzo HA: *An evaluation and treatment manual of osteopathic muscle energy procedures*, Valley Park, Mo, 1979, Mitchell, Moran and Pruzzo.
21. Ramirez MA, Haman J, Worth L: Low back pain: diagnosis by six newly discovered sacral tender points and treatment with counterstrain, *J Am Osteopath Assoc* 89:7, 1989.

22. Ramnurti M: *Fundamentals of yoga*, New York, 1972, Doubleday.
23. Rosomoff HL: Do herniated discs cause pain? *Clin J Pain* 1:91, 1985.
24. Rosomoff HL, Fishbain DA, Goldberg M, Steele-Rosomoff R: Physical findings in patients with chronic intractable benign pain of the neck and/or back, *Pain* 37:279, 1989.
25. Roth GB: *Counterstrain: positional release therapy* (study guide), Toronto, 1992, Wellness Institute, self-published.
26. Roth GB: Towards a unified model of musculoskeletal dysfunction. Presented at Canadian Chiropratic Association annual meeting, June, 1995.
27. Rumney IC: Structural diagnosis and manipulative therapy, *J Osteopathy* 70:21, 1963.
28. Schiowitz S: Facilitated positional release, *J Am Osteopath Assoc* 2:145, 1990.
29. Schwartz HR: The use of counterstrain in an acutely ill in-hospital population, *J Am Osteopath Assoc* 86:433, 1986.
30. Schwartz JS: *Human energy systems*, New York, 1980, Dutton.
31. Smith FF: *Inner bridges: a guide to energy movement and body structure*, Atlanta, 1986, Humanics.
32. Sutherland WG: The cranial bowl, *J Am Osteopath Assoc* 2:348, 1944.
33. Travell JG, Simons DG: *Myofascial pain and dysfunction: the trigger point manual*, Baltimore, 1983, Williams & Wilkins.
34. Weiselfish S: *Manual therapy for the orthopedic and neurologic patient emphasizing strain and counterstrain technique*, Hartford, Conn, 1993, Regional Physical Therapy, self-published.
35. Woodroffe J: *The serpent power*, Madras, India, 1918, Ganesh.
36. Woolerton H, McLean CJ: *Acupuncture energy in health and disease: a practical guide for advanced students*, Northamptonshire, England, 1979, Thorsons.

2

The Rationale for Positional Release Therapy

This chapter establishes a rational basis of understanding for the clinical phenomena associated with positional release therapy (PRT). Somatic dysfunction is discussed in the light of recent discoveries regarding the physiologic properties of the various tissues of the body. Several models of dysfunction are introduced within the context of their possible role in explaining the effects of PRT. Certain prevailing doctrines may be challenged by the arguments presented, and we hope that the reader will keep an open mind and judge these theories on their rational merit and on the basis of how they fit with clinical experience.

¶SOMATIC DYSFUNCTION

A NEW PARADIGM

Prevailing theories regarding the development of musculoskeletal conditions are undergoing intense scrutiny. Patients and insurers are demanding effectiveness and reliability in therapeutic intervention. If the underlying theory regarding the development of somatic dysfunction is inconsistent with clinical and physiologic realities, therapeutic models based on these principles must be questioned.

The structural model of musculoskeletal dysfunction is associated with gross anatomic and postural deformations and degenerative changes (scoliosis, disc degeneration, osteophytes, etc.). The presence of these physical anomalies are considered a direct cause of symptoms. These theories

have been supported by the advent of imaging devices such as the x-ray and its modern derivations (CT scan, MRI). The aim of therapies based on this model is to reshape the structure according to an architectural ideal. The assumption is that, by reestablishing the optimal physical relationship between body parts, everything will be restored to perfect working order. The therapeutic intervention is designed to remodel the components of the body and to relieve perceived structural stress within the system. Stretching shortened tissue, vigorously exercising hypotonic muscles and surgically refashioning osseous and articular components of the musculoskeletal system with the aim of achieving this architectural ideal have had limited success. The belief that these procedures should work because they are consistent with this model of the body encourages persistence, even though the objective results may contradict the underlying premise.[17,18,45] Unfortunately, in many cases, the structure resists our efforts. The result is often frustration for the practitioner and torment for the patient.

The functional model of the musculoskeletal system holds that biomechanical disturbances are a manifestation of the intrinsic properties of the tissues affected.[33] The tissue changes may be the result of trauma or inflammation and are seen as a direct expression of fundamental processes at the ultrastructural and biochemical levels. These changes, which are collectively referred to as somatic dysfunction, may be expressed as reduced joint play; loss of tissue resilience, tone, or elasticity; temperature and trophic changes; and loss of overt range of motion and postural asymmetry. This model views the form of the body as an expression of its function. Posture is seen as an outward manifestation of the degree of balance within the tissues, and greater emphasis is placed on the interaction of all of the body parts during physiologic and nonphysiologic motion. This model emphasizes the role of the soft tissues, especially the myofascial elements.

A growing body of knowledge supports the premise that a large proportion of musculoskeletal pain and dysfunction arises from the myofascial elements as opposed to neural or articular tissues.[38] Rosomoff and others[35] have concluded that over 90% of all back pain may be myofascial in origin. In fact, they contend that one of the most popular theories for the origin of back pain, that of pressure on a nerve, as in disk degeneration or disk protrusion, would result in a so-called silent nerve. They state that "back pain must be considered to be a non-surgical problem, unrelated to neural compression." Pressure on a nerve results in reduced sensation and motor function, not pain. This can easily be proven by the common experience of placing the arm on the back of a chair and noting how the arm "falls asleep." During this episode, there is a sensation of numbness and loss of motor control—not pain. It is only when the pressure is relieved that pain is experienced, along with the gradual return of motor function.

Saal and others[38] have proposed that, when disks are injured or are in the process of degeneration, they release water and proteoglycans. This material undergoes biochemical transformation through glycosylation and is subsequently targeted by the immune system as a foreign substance. This results in the initiation of an inflammatory response. As the leakage of this "foreign" protein into the epidural space continues, there may be a significant rise in the levels of phopholipase (a component of the arachadonic cascade), leading to the production of nociceptive chemical mediators and biochemically induced pain.[38] Brown[5] notes that disk herniations may be a "red herring" in many cases of thoracic pain and that, barring any significant indications of spinal cord compression, a conservative approach to relieving the myofascial source of the pain is all that is required.

Rosomoff and others[35] point out that, in most cases of musculoskeletal trauma, the accompanying soft tissue injury and the resulting release of inflammatory chemical mediators produce the sensation of pain. Myofascial responses to injury result from an increased level of proinflammatory chemicals present because of the injury or from direct trauma to the tissues.[49] In the latter case it is postulated that calcium is released from the disrupted muscle, which in turn combines with adenosine triphosphate to produce sustained contracture.[7] Proprioceptive and neuromuscular responses are other potentially important mechanisms associated with somatic dysfunction. The sudden strain that accompanies many injuries engages the myotatic reflex arc.[22,53] These events may account for the development of myofascial trigger points, protective muscle spasm, reduced range of motion, and decreased muscle strength, which consistently accompany musculoskeletal injury.

The effect of trauma to the fascial matrix is also a subject of much speculation. The discoveries of Levin[27-29] may shed some light on this complex issue. He and others have demonstrated that the underlying structure of all organic tissue determines its responses to traumatic forces and may account for certain properties that can lead to persisting dysfunction.[19,36,51]

PRT, and other functional therapies, do not alleviate or attempt to treat any tissue pathology. The primary role of these therapies is to relieve the somatic dysfunction, which, according to Levin,[29] is a *nonlinear* process. A nonlinear process is one that exerts an influence over a relatively brief period of time. These processes tend to be functional rather than pathologic and respond rapidly to functional therapy. Functional restoration establishes an environment in which the *linear* healing process of the pathologic component of the injury may occur more efficiently.

Musculoskeletal dysfunction therefore appears to originate and be maintained at the molecular and ultrastructural level within the tissues. The intrinsic properties of tissue and their inherent pathophysiologic response to trauma seem to be consistent with many of the external manifestations associated with somatic dysfunction. It is imperative that we examine our beliefs and hypotheses so that we can accommodate this developing knowledge base within our working model of somatic dysfunction. Effective therapy must be congruent with these principles regarding the response of the body tissues to trauma. We will now examine PRT within the context of its influence on these properties of tissue.

THE TISSUES

The body is composed of several major tissue types. For the purposes of this discussion, with respect to musculoskeletal dysfunction, we will consider three main classes of tissue: muscle, fascia, and bone. Even though these tissues are considered separately and are often discussed in isolation from each other in the literature, we should recognize that they are interconnected functionally. The *kinetic chain* theory[14] and the *tensegrity* model of the body[27-29] support the concept that the effects associated with somatic lesions are transmitted throughout the organism. Restriction or dysfunction in one area or type of tissue can result in reactions and symptoms in other areas of the body. Effective musculoskeletal therapy, including PRT, should address the source of the dysfunction, and thus it is essential to have a thorough understanding of the physiology and pathophysiology of the somatic tissues.

The muscular system, despite its massive proportions, is maintained in a subtle state of balance and coordination throughout a wide range of postures and activities. The muscles are the source and the recipient of the greatest amount of neural activity in the body. This includes sensory and motor activity, vertical (conscious, cerebral) pathways, and autonomic activity in relation to the metabolic, visceral, and circulatory demands required during muscular exertion. The muscles, according to Janda, are "at the crossroads of afferent and efferent stimuli" and are, in fact, "the most exposed part of the motor system."[22] Range of motion, segmentally and globally, is largely dependent on the state of balance of the muscles that cross the involved joints, and restriction of motion may be directly attributed to abnormalities in the tone and activity of this system.

The response of muscle to injury is *protective muscle spasm*, and this reflex is mediated by local proprioceptors and monosynaptic reflexes at the spinal level. The neuromuscular reflexes involved in this response will be discussed in greater detail later in this chapter in the section on proprioceptors. Muscle is interwoven with collagenous and elastic fibers and therefore shares certain characteristics with fascial tissue. Fibrous tissue changes within the muscle may thus be a feature of posttraumatic dysfunction.

The fascial system is a vast network of fibrous tissue that contains and supports muscles, viscera, and other tissues throughout the body. Injury or inflammation results in adhesive fibrogenesis, which may result in the loss of normal elasticity. According to Barnes[1] and Becker,[3] the collagenous matrix of the fascia is in a state of dynamic adaptation to changing conditions, including the effects of strain, trauma, and inflammatory processes. Fascia contains a higher percentage of inelastic collagen fibers than elastin fibers and thus plays an important role in limiting excessive motion and containing inflammation and infection. Alterations in the electrochemical bonds between collagen fibers results in the formation of cross-linkages in response to chemical irritation related to inflammation, overstretch, or other mechanical influences. As these cross-linkages form, the elasticity of the fascia becomes reduced and the tissue alters from a *sol* to a *gel* state within the area of involvement. The net effect is the development of an area of restriction and reduced elasticity, or *fascial tension*.[1,35] Neural tension and visceral dysfunction have also been cited as separate foci of dysfunction.[2,6] These lesions may represent specific manifestations of fascial tension within these tissues.

Osseous structures have long been ignored as active elements in the pathophysiology of musculoskeletal dysfunction. Recent evidence indicates that bone is much more plastic and responsive than had been previously appreciated. Chauffour[11] states that fresh long bone has flexibility of up to 30 degrees before the induction of fracture. The collagenous matrix of bone and the periosteum exhibit characteristics similar to fascia elsewhere in the body. In an injury, bone is no less affected than any other component of the musculoskeletal system and will display persisting injury patterns depending on the nature of the event. Many of the therapeutic modalities used for muscle and fascia may, theoretically, be applied to the osseous component of the dysfunction.[10,42]

THE SIGNIFICANCE OF THE TENDER POINT

Tender points may arise in any of the somatic tissues: muscle, fascia (including ligaments, tendons, articular capsule, synchondroses, and cranial sutures), periosteum, and bone. The tender points in positional release therapy are used primarily as diagnostic indicators of the location of the dysfunction. The diagnostic and therapeutic utilization of tender points is central to a wide range of therapies, including PRT.* An understanding of their pathophysiology and role in the etiology of somatic dysfunction will help us in pursuing our study of PRT.

Myofascial pain syndrome (MPS) is defined by Travell and Simons[45] as follows: "localized musculoskeletal pain originating from a hyperirritable spot or trigger point (TrP) within a taut band of skeletal muscle or muscle fascia." A thorough review of the literature with respect to MPS reveals a decided lack of objective criteria for evaluating and treating this common condition.[15] The tender point (TP) is palpable as a small (0.25 to 1.0 cm) nodule, usually located in the subcutaneous, muscular, or fascial tissues. There appears to be a close association between the tender points used in PRT and by Jones with the Ah Shi points as described in Chinese writings,[8] the neurolymphatic points as described by Chapman and Owens,[9] and the neurovascular points described by Bennett.[4] (See Chapter 1.)

The association of myofascial trigger points or tender points with musculoskeletal dysfunction has been established by numerous authors.† Sedentary lifestyles and occupational repetitiveness limit the number of muscles used on a regular basis. Therefore a relatively small percentage of our total muscle mass tends to be overworked, while other muscles become atrophied and reduced in their ability to tolerate loads or strain. Postural stress, trauma, articular strain, and other mechanical factors may excessively load myofascial tissues, leading to the biochemical changes involved in the production of TPs. Tender points are most prevalent in mechanically stressed tissues, notably those subject to increased postural demands, such as the upper trapezius, the levator scapula, the suboccipitals, the psoas, and the quadratus lumborum.[30] On deeper palpation, the intrinsic muscles of the axial skeleton (the multifidus, rotatores, levator costorum, scalene, and intercostal muscles) are also often found to contain active TPs. The "weekend warrior" often strains the underused muscle groups and demands phasic responses from muscles which have adapted to a primarily tonic function.

Inflammation caused by the initiating injury releases proinflammatory and vasoconstrictive chemical mediators such as histamine and prostaglandins. Acute or repetitive

---

*References 8, 22, 31, 35, 39, 42, 45, 48.
†References 15, 20, 35, 41, 45, 46, 54-57. 58

trauma may result in the rupturing of the sarcoplasmic reticulum. The ensuing flood of calcium ions into the interstitial compartment leads to uncontrolled actin and myosin interaction and the development of the palpable taut bands of muscle associated with myofascial involvement. The result of these traumatic events is hypertonicity, inflammation, ischemia, and an increased concentration of metabolically active chemical mediators. This vicious cycle, which will be further perpetuated by repetitive trauma, is thought to be responsible for the maintenance of these hyperirritable, constricted focal areas of inflammation (TPs) within the tissues.[23,43,49]

Sensitization of nociceptive and mechanoreceptive organs within the affected tissues appears to have a role in mediating the formation TPs. Group III and IV nerve fibers are sensitive to chemically active compounds such as prostaglandins, kinins, histamine, and potassium. Microscopic examination of muscular TPs reveals the presence of mast cells (source of histamine) and platelets (source of serotonin). These proinflammatory substances may contribute to the local hypersensitivity that activates the TPs when mechanical deformation or direct pressure occurs.[43]

The myofascial tissues are, in essence, a continuous network that surrounds and penetrates all of the structures and organs of the body without interruption. This can be compared with a piece of woven fabric or a net. Any disruption, pressure, or kink within this net is instantaneously transmitted to the entire structure and will create a distortion of the previously symmetric architecture.[15,27,34] The tender point may be conceived of as a focus of constriction of the myofascial tissues. These nodular focal points of tension (TPs) within the myofascial continuum may result in distortions in the biomechanical integrity of this matrix.[1] They may also play a role in generating irritable stimuli, which maintain the dysfunction via a facilitated segment (discussed later).

THE ROLE OF POSITIONAL RELEASE THERAPY IN SOMATIC DYSFUNCTION

The role of PRT in the resolution of somatic dysfunction is assessed within the context of several of the current theories of myofascial and neuromuscular pathophysiology. Each of these processes may explain a certain aspect of the dysfunction, and a combination of effects may account for the range of manifestations found in clinical practice.

POSITIONAL RELEASE THERAPY TREATMENT

Positional release therapy treatment is accomplished by placing the involved tissues in an ideal position of comfort (POC). The purpose of the POC is to reduce the irritability of the tender point and to normalize the tissues associated with the dysfunction. Precision is required in positioning the patient because the range within which the maximal relaxation of tissues occurs is small—usually 2

to 3 degrees.[22] (See Chapter 4.) It may be speculated that positioning beyond this ideal range places the antagonistic muscles or opposing fascial structures under increased stretch, which in turn causes a proprioceptive/neural spillover, resulting in reactivation of the facilitated segment. The ideal position is determined subjectively by the patient's perception of tenderness and objectively by the reduction in palpable tone of the tender point. We refer to this change as the comfort zone (CZ). This intrinsic feedback system assists in the diagnosis and treatment of musculoskeletal dysfunction and affords PRT a high level of reliability within the clinical setting.

D'Ambrogio and Weiselfish, in their lectures, describe two major phases of the release phenomenon: the neuromuscular phase, which lasts approximately 90 seconds, and the myofascial phase, which may last for up to 20 minutes. Weiselfish[53] further states that the neuromuscular phase in neurologic patients usually lasts for approximately 3 minutes. (See Chapter 1.) Clinically, several phenomena occur during the positioning. As one approaches the CZ, the tissues in the area of the tender point soften and become less tender. After a period of time, several other observations may be noted. There is often an increase in local temperature. Vibration and pulsation in the area of the tender point are also common findings as the treatment progresses. The breath may be observed to alter during the session, becoming shallow and rapid, followed by several slow, deep breaths. This may occur several times during the treatment. Fascial unwinding may be sensed extending from the area of the tender point. The patient often reports several transient symptoms during the course of the positioning, including paresthesia, sensation of heat, fleeting pains in other areas of the body, headaches, emotional episodes, and ultimately, a sense of deep relaxation.

The observed phenomena associated with somatic dysfunction and the therapeutic effect of PRT may be explained by several pathophysiological mechanisms: proprioceptive systems, nociceptive pathways, the facilitated segment, and fascial dysfunction.

PROPRIOCEPTORS: NEUROMUSCULAR FEEDBACK

In the 1940s Denslow[12] and Korr[25,26] began investigating the role of neuromuscular feedback systems in the development of somatic dysfunction. In functional technic, as described by Hoover,[18] range of motion is monitored for the degree of *ease* or *bind*. He describes a lesion as having an excessively resistant range of motion in one direction and an excessively compliant range in another direction. These characteristics are not ascribed to any particular tissue. Jones[22] is specific in describing his technique as the placing of the body in the direction of greatest ease or comfort to "arrest inappropriate proprioceptor activity."

The proprioceptive organs that monitor the musculoskeletal system are located in three major areas. The Ruffini receptors are found in the joint capsule and report

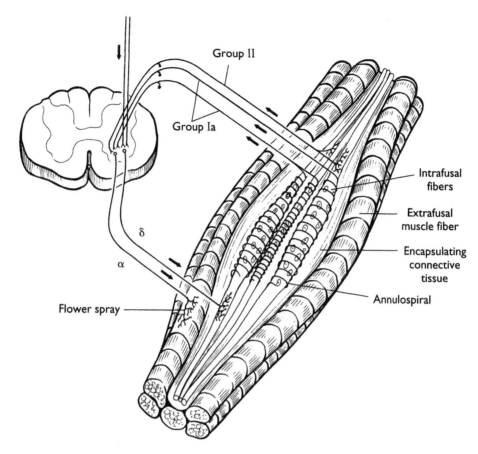

Fig. 2-1 *Muscle spindle and spinal segment.*

position, velocity, and direction of motion. This information is transmitted directly to higher centers in the cerebellum and the cerebral cortex and do not seem to have any direct influence at the local segmental level. The Golgi tendon organs are located near the musculotendinous junction and respond to excessive tension and load on the muscle. Impulses from these receptors exert an inhibitory effect at the spinal level to protect the tissues from overstretch. The muscle spindles are located between the muscle fibers of all striated muscle. The monitoring system of this complex organelle is discussed later.[25,48,50]

The muscle spindles are perhaps the most sensitive of the proprioceptive organs to the moment-to-moment changes in position, load, and velocity of body parts (Fig. 2-1). They are connected, directly and indirectly, to the spinal segment by gamma and alpha motor neurons, which supply the intrafusal (muscle spindle) fibers and the extrafusal (somatic muscle) fibers, respectively. Two types of receptors within the muscle spindle generate afferent impulses. The *flower spray* endings located near the ends of the spindles are stimulated by the degree of stretch on the intrafusal fibers (type II sensory neurons). The annulospiral endings, located around the central nuclear bag of the intrafusal fibers, report not only degree of stretch, but also the rate of

change of length (type Ia sensory neurons). The velocity of change of length has great significance in that it is a predictive stimulus for potential injury to the muscle and related tissues. This critical aspect of the sensory function of the muscle spindle appears to predominate in terms of neural influence at the spinal level. Thus a force that produces a rapid change in length, such as a sudden stretch on a muscle, will have a more powerful effect in generating protective reflexes via the monosynaptic connection to the alpha motor neuron. The gamma efferent neurons determine the length of the intrafusal fibers and establish the threshold for stimulation of the sensory neurons. A predetermined resting tone, or *gamma bias*, is maintained to ensure the ability of the somatic muscles to respond to changing demands. The dynamic balance between the muscle spindle and somatic muscle as mediated by the gamma system has been referred to as a high-gain servomechanism.[25,26] This system maintains ideal tone and preparedness of the muscle and may also be a mechanism for the development and perpetuation of the response to myofascial injury.

According to Jones,[22] the muscle spindle apparatus plays a predominant role in the development of somatic dysfunction. In his book, Jones describes the effect of a strain on a pair of antagonistic muscles (A and B) on a joint. Figure 2-2,

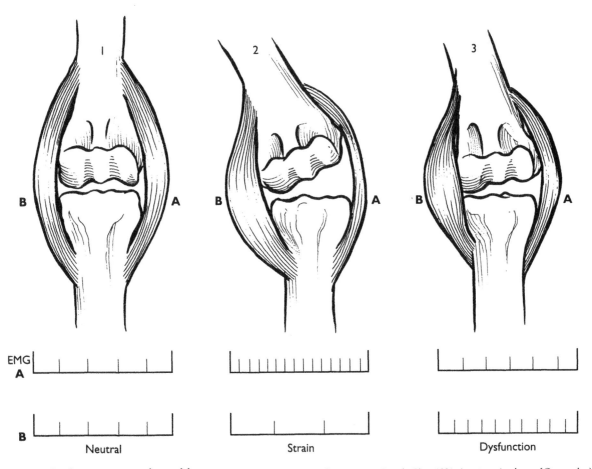

Fig. 2-2 *Jones neuromuscular model.* (Modified from Jones LH: *Strain and counterstrain,* Newark, Ohio, 1981, American Academy of Osteopathy.)

which is divided into three sections, illustrates this theory. Section 1 represents a joint at rest with approximately an equal state of tone within both muscles, as displayed in the electromyogram (EMG) schematic. Section 2 shows a condition of joint strain. Muscle A is overstretched, causing an increased rate of neural impulses to be generated within the gamma system. Muscle B is in a hypershortened state, resulting in a decreased rate of impulses. The sudden stretch that occurs in muscle A results in a myotatic reflex contraction and a rapid rebound from the initial direction of strain. This produces a sudden stretching of the hypershortened muscle B. The annulospiral endings, which respond mainly to the rate of change of length, would theoretically be hyperstimulated as muscle B is suddenly stretched, resulting in the generation of a massive neural discharge in relation to this muscle. Section 3 represents the joint subsequent to the injury. It is unable to return to neutral because of the hypershortened state of muscle B.[22] Thus muscle B may become a primary source of the persisting dysfunction.

This explanation may account for one aspect of the dysfunction, and in theory it is at this level that PRT may exert a major influence during the initial 90-second interval (approximately 3 minutes for the neurologic patient). The POC, by moving away from the restriction barrier and in the direction of greatest ease, essentially reduces the tension on the affected tissues and minimizes the stimulation of the affected proprioceptors. By some mechanism, as yet not understood, maintaining the POC for a minimum period of approximately 90 seconds appears to neutralize this otherwise nonadapting reflex arc, which is responsible for the continuing hypertonicity. This theory, however, fails to explain some of the other observed effects associated with somatic dysfunction.

NOCICEPTORS: PAIN PATHWAYS

Tissue injury is accompanied by the release of arachadonic acid. This initiates the so-called arachadonic cascade and results in the production of prostaglandin, thromboxane, monohydroxy fatty acids, and leukotrienes, which promotes the progression of the inflammatory response and the development of hyperalgesia. This in turn results in vasodilation, the attraction of leukocytes, the release of complement activators, and the release of pain-producing neuropeptides such as histamine, serotonin, and bradykinin.[24,32,49,52]

Van Buskirk[48] makes a compelling argument for the role of the small myelinated (type III) and unmyelinated (type IV) peripheral neurons, which constitute the nociceptive system and which respond directly to the chemical mediators associated with tissue trauma and hypoxia. These free

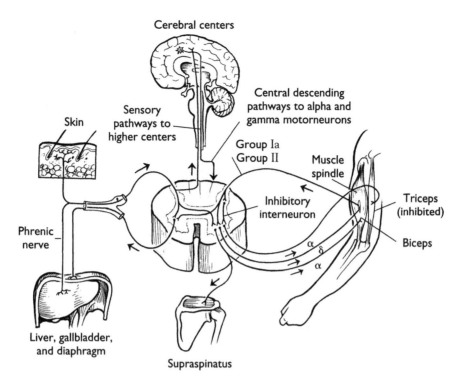

Fig. 2-3 *Facilitated segment components (C5-7).*

nerve endings are distributed throughout all of the connective tissues of the body with the exception of the stroma of the brain. These receptors are stimulated by neuropeptides produced by noxious influences, including trauma, chemical irritation, metabolic or visceral disturbance, or pathology. Impulses generated in these neurons spread centrally and also peripherally along the numerous branches of each neuron. At the terminus of the axons, peptide neurotransmitters such as substance P are released. The response of the musculoskeletal system to these painful stimuli may thus play a central role in the development of somatic dysfunction.

According to Van Buskirk[48] and Schmidt,[40] nociceptors are known to produce muscle guarding reactions and the autonomic changes associated with somatic dysfunction. Because proprioceptors are not present in all of the tissues that may be connected with somatic dysfunction (bone, viscera), the role of nociceptors should be considered as potential agents in the perpetuation of the irritable reflexes associated with these conditions.

The action of PRT on the nociceptive system may be exerted through the relaxation of the surrounding tissues and the resulting improvement in vascular and interstitial circulation. This may have an indirect effect on removing the chemical mediators of inflammation. The subsequent resolution of the guarding reflexes in the myofascial structures may also contribute to a reduction in the release of further nociceptive substances. Postional release therapy may also act on this traumatic cycle by helping to resolve "facilitated segments" within the central nervous system.

THE FACILITATED SEGMENT: NEURAL CROSSROADS

In 1947, Denslow and Korr[12] introduced the concept of the facilitated segment and described it as follows:

> A lesion represents a facilitated segment of the spinal cord, maintained in that state by impulses of endogenous origin entering the corresponding dorsal root. All structures receiving efferent nerve fibers from that segment are, therefore, potentially exposed to excessive excitation or inhibition.

The central nervous system (CNS) is continuously subject to afferent impulses arising from countless reporting stations (receptors) throughout the body. Within any given segment of the spinal cord, there are a fixed number of sensory and motor neurons. Much like the relay centers in a telephone exchange, there are limits to the number of "calls" that can be handled. If the number or amplitude of impulses from the proprioceptors, nociceptors, and higher centers channeled to a particular segment exceeds the capacity of the normal routing pathway, the electrochemical discharges may begin to affect collateral pathways. This spillover effect may be exerted ipsilaterally, contralaterally, or vertically. Impulses may arise from any tissue (fascia, muscle, articular capsule, meninges, viscera, skin, cerebral cognitive or emotional centers, etc.). When these impulses extend beyond their normal sensorimotor pathways, the CNS begins to misinterpret the information because of the effect of an overflow of neurotransmitter substance within the involved segment. For example, afferent impulses intended to register as pain in the gallbladder manifest as shoulder pain. The phrenic nerve and portions of the brachial plexus share common spinal origins. This may also be the basis of so-called referred pain.[32]

The resulting overload at the CNS level is referred to as a facilitated segment (FS) (Fig. 2-3). Chronic irritation can involve the sympathetic/autonomic pathways and lead to trophic and metabolic changes, which may be the basis for some of the local tissue changes associated with musculoskeletal dysfunction. The neuromuscular reflex arc is at the crossroads for several sources of noxious stimuli, including trauma, viscerosomatic reflexes, and emotional distress, as well as the vast proprioceptive system reporting from striated muscle throughout the body. According to Upledger,[47] the facilitated segment is exemplified by the following:

1. *Hypersensitivity.* Minimal impulses may produce excessive responses or sensations because of a reduced threshold for stimulation and depolarization at the level of the FS.
2. *Overflow.* Impulses may become nonspecific and spill over to adjacent pathways. Collateral nerve cells, lateral tracts, and vertical tracts may be stimulated and produce symptoms of a widely divergent nature. Referred pain may be produced.
3. *Autonomic dystrophy.* The sympathetic ganglia become excessively activated, leading to reduced healing and repair of target cells, reduced immune function, impaired circulation, accelerated aging, and deterioration of peripheral tissues. Digestive and cardiovascular disturbances and visceral parenchymal dystrophy may also develop over time.

Because of the excessive discharge arising from a variety of receptors, the facilitated segment may eventually become a self-perpetuating source of irritation in its own right. An injury, for example, of the biceps produces an increase in high-frequency discharge (increased neural impulses), which is transmitted by way of the type Ia and II neurons, to the spinal segment at the level of C5. If the discharge is excessive, other muscles connected to this segment (supraspinatus, teres minor, levator scapula, pectoralis minor, etc.) may receive a certain amount of spillover discharge. This results in an increase in the gamma gain to these muscles. Thus several muscles supplied by the same segment may have a generally increased setting of their gamma bias (background tone fed to the muscle spindle apparatus), which leads to increased hypertonicity and susceptibility to strain. Other tissues (skin receptors, viscera, and cerebral emotional centers) may also feed into this loop either as primary sources of high-frequency discharge or secondary to the neuromuscularly induced hyperirritability.[50]

Positional release therapy appears to have a damping influence on the general level of excitability within the facilitated segment. Weiselfish[53] has found that this characteristic of PRT is unique in its effectiveness and has utilized this feature to successfully treat severe neurologic patients even though the source of the primary dysfunction arose from the supraspinal level. Postional release therapy appears

to exert an influence in reducing the threshold within the FS and may thus open a window of opportunity for the CNS to normalize the level of neural activity.[48]

FASCIAL DYSFUNCTION: CONNECTIVE TISSUE CONNECTIONS

In the late 1970s, Stephen Levin, an orthopedic surgeon, conceived of a model for the structure of organic tissue that could account for many physical and clinical characteristics. Through a process of systematic evaluation of the basic physical properties of tissue, he arrived at the conclusion that all organic tissue must be composed of a type of truss (triangular form) and that the essential building block of all tissue must be the *tension icosohedron*.[27-29] This model, also referred to as the *tensegrity model* and the *myofascial skeletal truss*, has gradually emerged as a viable explanation for the nature of organic tissue. Recently, this model has been confirmed by electron-microscopic methods and through physical stress extrapolation experiments.[19,51] This model accounts for the concept of the *kinetic chain*, which recognizes that lesions transmit tensions throughout the body and that symptoms can be traced back to their source and treated indirectly by aligning fascial lines of force in relation to the primary focus of restriction (Fig. 2-4).[14,34]

The implications of Levin's model, from a clinical perspective, are that all tissues share certain fundamental characteristics. Indeed, this model confirms that all tissues are alike at the molecular and ultrastructural level. The tension icosohedron helps clarify the properties of the tissues and may be predictive of the effects of any therapeutic system. The tensegrity model delineates the following properties of somatic tissue: the forces maintaining the structure of the body are tension and compression and have no bending moments (such as in the hinge mechanism ascribed to joints); the structural integrity of the body is gravity independent and is stable with flexible joints; the tissues of the body have a nonlinear stress/strain response to external forces; and the body is a functional unit, in that forces applied to it at one point are transmitted uniformly and instantaneously throughout the entire organism.

This model implies that a perceived condition in one area of the body may have its origin in another area and that therapeutic action at the source of the dysfunction will have an immediate, corrective effect on all secondary areas, including the site of symptom manifestation. It also may account for some of the physiologic effects that produce the release phenomenon.[1]

Because of this interconnectedness of the entire fascial system, restriction in one area may result in a reduced range of motion in a distal structure.[3,10,14] The area of perception of pain by the patient, especially in chronic cases, may often be remote from the area of the most sensitive tender points. Because the tender points represent areas of relative fixation, these areas are, in essence, *splinted,* and this results in lines of tension that extend to peripheral structures. As we move peripherally from the primary focus of restriction, the reduce the excessive tissue play and range of motion. Therapies such as fusion or prolotherapy create relative fixation of tissues.[13] The reduced mechanical strain and the consequent diminishment in the release of nociceptive mediators result in reduced pain. These approaches may, however, also produce secondary lesions and an increase in aberrant biomechanics.

It is hypothesized that PRT, by reducing the tension on the myofascial system, also engages the fascial components of the dysfunction. The reduction in tension on the collagenous cross-linkages appears to induce a disengagement of the electrochemical bonds and a conversion back to the *sol* state. This fascial component of release during the POC appears to require a maintenance of the positioning for several minutes. The 90 second interval espoused by Jones theoretically addresses only the neuromuscular aspect of the dysfunction.

Some of the effects of the POC may be directly attributable to the changes in the condition of the fascial matrix itself. Others may be due to autonomic and electrochemical associations between the myofascial structures and other systems.[42] The resulting reduction in tension at the level of the primary lesion would, in accordance with the tensegrity model, create an equilibration of tension throughout the organism. The previous discrepancy between hypomobile and hypermobile areas would be resolved, and there would be a reduction in the abnormal biomechanical stresses associated with the stimulation of pain receptors.

Positional release therapy thus appears to be capable of initiating a release of tension patterns both at the neuromuscular level and at the fascial level. The determining factors are the precision and skill exercised by the practitioner in maintaining the ideal position and the length of time required for the completion of the release process.

⁊ SUMMARY

New paradigms are emerging that are more consistent with clinical observation in the field of musculoskeletal dysfunction. Current models recognize the intrinsic properties of the tissues and how these are affected at the ultrastructural level. Somatic dysfunction may manifest within any of the tissues of the body. Each of these tissues expresses trauma and dysfunction in unique ways and is interconnected with all of the tissues of the body as part of a kinetic chain. Thus trauma to one part of the body may result in persisting dysfunction in any other part.

The tender point is a clinically recognized expression of somatic dysfunction and is used in PRT as a diagnostic indicator.

Several pathophysiologic mechanisms may be responsible for the development of the clinical manifestations associated with somatic dysfunction. Neuromuscular responses, mediated by monosynaptic reflexes and musculotendinous proprioceptors, can alter the length/tension relationship of the muscular component of the dysfunction. Tissue injury results in the release of proinflammatory

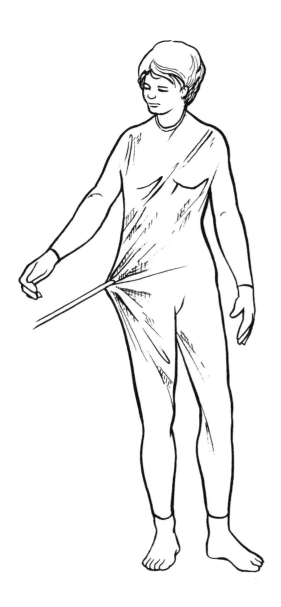

Fig. 2-4 *Representation of fascial tension patterns.*

tensegrity structure of the tissues transmits these forces, without any loss of intensity, to an area of the body which interfaces with external mechanical influences.

The body attempts to create a full range of gross motion by compensating for areas of relative fixation. This results in excessive motion in regions of the body that extend from the focus of dysfunction. Excessive force, due to strain or repetitive motion against the restriction barrier, may cause local inflammation and pain. The increased mechanical deformation and stretch within these tissues may result in the release of pain-producing chemical mediators. Thus pain may be expressed within tissues, which are, in fact, secondary areas of involvement. The goal of treatment of these hypermobile tissues (joints, ligaments, etc.) is to chemical mediators, which in turn stimulate the pain receptors within the involved tissues. This further promotes the development and maintenance of protective muscle spasm and may result in a persisting dysfunction, which can become a focal point for reinjury and continuing pain. This cycle of events feeds into the neurologic phenomenon referred to as the facilitated segment. Other, nonsomatic stimuli may also interact with this pathway and lead to a self-perpetuating cycle of irritability. Fascial structures respond to trauma and the ensuing inflammatory process through the production of adhesive cross-fibers and fascial tension, which may impair mobility throughout the organism. The tensegrity model of organic tissue has given new insight into the nature of tissue interactions and a greater understanding of the pathophysiology of somatic dysfunction.

Positional release therapy theoretically addresses neuromuscular hyperirritability and muscular hypertonicity as mediated by the proprioceptive system. It also appears to reduce tissue tension, allowing for the resolution of the inflammatory response and the release of the electrochemical bonds associated with fascial restriction. Any tissue may be implicated in the pathophysiology of somatic dysfunction. The clinician should be guided by tissue response rather than by symptoms in the search for the underlying cause and treatment of the dysfunction.

References

1. Barnes J: *Myofascial release: the search for excellence*, 1990, self-published.
2. Barral JP: *Visceral manipulation*, Seattle, 1988, Eastland Press.
3. Becker RF: The meaning of fascia and fascial continuity, *Osteopathic Ann*, 1975:35-46.
4. Bennett R: In Chapman's Reflexes. Martin R. editor: *Dynamics of correction of abnormal function*, Sierre Madre, Calif, 1977, self-published.
5. Brown CW: Change in disc treatment saves hockey star, *Back Let* 7(12):1, 1992.
6. Butler DS: *Mobilisation of the nervous system*, Melbourne, 1991, Churchill Livingstone.
7. Caillet R: *Soft tissue pain and disability*, Philadelphia, 1980, Davis.
8. Chaitow L: *The acupuncture treatment of pain*, Wellingborough, 1976, Thorsons.
9. Chapman F, Owens C: *Introduction to and endocrine interpretation of chapman's reflexes*, self-published.
10. Chauffour P: *Lien mechanique* (mechanical link), Paris, 1986, Maloine.
11. Chauffour P: Lectures (mechanical link), Palm Beach, FL, 1994, 1995.
12. Denslow JS, Korr IM, Krems AB: Quanitative studies of chronic facilitation in human motoneuron pool. *Am J Physiol* 150:229, 1947.
13. Dorman TA, editor: Prolotherapy in the lumbar spine and pelvis, *Spine: state of the Art Reviews* 9(2), May 1995.
14. Gray G: Functional kinetic chain rehabilitation: overuse and inflammatory conditions and their management, *Sports Medicine Update*, 1993.
15. Henriksson KG: Microscopic and biochemical changes in fibromyalgia, *Proc 1st Int Symp MP* May 1989 (abstract).
16. Hey LR, Helewa A: Myofascial pain syndrome: a critical review of the literature, *J Can Phys Assoc* 46:28, 1994.
17. Hey LR, Helewa A: The effects of stretch and spray on women with myofascial pain syndrome: a pilot study, *Physiother Can*, 44:4, 1992 (abstract).
18. Hoover HV: Functional technic, *AAO Year Book* 47, 1958.
19. Imgber DE, Jamieson J: Cells as tensegrity structures: architectural regulation of histodifferentiation by physical forces transduced over basement membrane. In Andersonn LL, Gahm CT, Kblom PE, editors: *Gene expression during normal and malignant differentiation*, New York, 1985, Academic Press.
20. Jaeger B, Reeves JL: Quantification of changes in myofascial trigger point sensitivity with the pressure algometer following passive stretch, *Pain* 27(2):203, 1986.
21. Janda V: Muscle and joint correlations. Proceedings, IV FINN, Prague, 1974, Rehabilitation Suppl 10-11, 154-158, 1975.
22. Jones LH: *Strain and counterstrain*, Newark, Ohio, 1981, American Academy of Osteopathy.
23. Kalyan-Raman UP and others: Muscle pathology in primary fibromyalgia syndrome: a light microscopic, histochemical and ultrastructural study, *J Rheumatol* 2:808, 1984.
24. Kanaka R, Schaible HG, Schmidt RF: Activation of fine articular afferent units by bradykinin, *Brain Res* 327:81, 1985.
25. Korr IM: Proprioceptors and the behaviour of lesioned segments, *Osteopath Ann* 2:12, 1974.
26. Korr IM: Proprioceptors and somatic dysfunction, *J Am Osteopath Assoc* 74:638, 1975.
27. Levin SM: The icosohedron as the three-dimensional finite element in biomechanical support. Proceedings of the Society of General Systems Research on Mental Images, Values and Reality, Philadelphia, Society of General Systems Research, May 1986.
28. Levin, SM: The space truss as a model for cervical spine mechanics—a systems science concept. In Paterson JK, Burn L, editors: *Back pain: an international review*, Boston, 1990, Kluwer Academic.
29. Levin SM: The importance of soft tissue for structural support of the body, *Spine: state of the art reviews*, 9(2):357, 1995.
30. Lowe JC: Treatment-resistant myofascial pain syndrome. In Hammer WI, editor: *Functional soft tissue examination and treatment by manual methods*, Gaithersburg, Md, 1991, Aspen.
31. Melzack R, Stillwell DM, Fex EJ: Trigger points and acupuncture points for pain: correlations and implications, *Pain* 3:3, 1977.
32. Mense S: Nervous outflow from skeletal muscle following chemical noxious stimulation, *J Physiol* 267:75, 1977.
33. Paris SV: Manual therapy: treat function not pain. In Michel TH, editor: *Pain*, New York, 1985, Churchill Livingstone.
34. Rolf I: *Rolfing, the integration of human structure*, New York, 1977, Harper & Row.
35. Rosomoff HL and others: Physical findings in patients with chronic intractable benign pain of the neck and/or back, *Pain* 37:279, 1989.
36. Roth GB: Towards a unified model of musculoskeletal dysfunction. Presented at Canadian Chiropractic Association annual meeting, June 1995.
37. Ruch TC: Pathophysiology of pain. In Ruch T, Patton HD, editors: *Physiology and biophysics: the brain and neural function*, ed 2, Philadelphia, 1979, Saunders.
38. Saal JS and others: Biochemical evidence of inflammation in discogenic lumbar radiculopathy: analysis of phospholipase

A2 activity in human herniated disc. In Proceedings of the International Society for Study of the Lumbar Spine, Kyoto, Japan, 1989.

39. Sarno JE: *Mind over back pain*, New York, 1982, Berkley.
40. Schmidt RF, Kniffki KD, Schomberg ED: Der Einfuss Klein Kalibriger Muskelafferenzen auf den Muskeltonus. In Bauer HJ and others: *Therapie der Spastik*, 1981, Verlag fur ange-wandte Wissenschaften, Munchen.
41. Scudds RA, Ewart NK, Traschel L: The treatment of myofascial trigger points with helium-neon and gallium-arsenide laser: a blinded, crossover trial, *Pain* 5(suppl):768, 1990 (abstract).
42. Smith FF: *Inner bridges: a guide to energy movement and body structure*, Atlanta, 1986, Humanics New Age.
43. Smolders JJ: Myofascial trigger points. In Hammer WI, editor: *Functional soft tissue examination and treatment by manual methods*, Gaithersburg, Md, 1991, Aspen.
44. Snow CJ and others: Randomized controlled clinical trial of stretch and spray for relief of back and neck myofascial pain, *Physiother Can* 44:8, 1992 (abstract).
45. Travell JG, Simons DG: *Myofascial pain and dysfunction: the trigger point manual*, Baltimore, 1983, Williams & Wilkins.
46. Travell JG, Rinzler SH: The myofascial genesis of pain, *Postgrad Med* 11:425, 1952.
47. Upledger JE: The facilitated segment, *Massage Ther J*, Summer 1989.
48. Van Buskirk RL: Nociceptive reflexes and the somatic dysfunction: a model, *J Am Osteopath Assoc* 9:792, 1990.
49. Vane JR: Pain of inflammation: an introduction. In Bonica J, Lindblom U, Iggo A, editors: *Advances in pain research and therapy*, vol 5, New York, 1983, Raven Press.
50. Wall PD: Physiological mechanisms involved in the production and relief of pain. In Bonica J, Procacci P, Pagni CA, editors: *Recent advances in pain: pathophysiological and clinical aspects*, Springfield, Ill, 1974, Charles C Thomas.
51. Wang N, Butler JP, Imgber DE: Mechanotransduction across the cell surface and through the cytoskeleton, *Science* 260:1124, 1993.
52. Weinstein JN: Anatomy and neurophysiologic mechanisms of spinal pain. In Frymoyer JW, editor: *The adult spine: principles and practice*, New York, 1991, Raven Press.
53. Weiselfish S: *Manual therapy for the orthopedic and neurologic patient emphasizing strain and counterstrain technique*, Hartford, Conn, 1993, Regional Physical Therapy, self-published.
54. Wolfe F: The clinical syndrome of fibrositis, *Am J Med* 81:7, 1986.
55. Wolfe F: Fibrositis, fibromyalgia and musculoskeletal disease: the current status of the fibrositis syndrome, *Arch Phys Med Rehab* 69:527, 1988.
56. Wolfe F and others: The fibromyalgia and myofascial pain syndromes: a preliminary study of tender points and trigger points in persons with fibromyalgia, myofascial pain syndrome and no disease, *J Rheumatol* 19(6):944, 1992.
57. Wolfe F and others: Criteria for fibromyalgia, *Arthritis Rheum* 32:S47, 1989.
58. Yunus MB and others: Pathological changes in muscle in primary fibromyalgia syndrome, *Am J Med* 81:38, 1986.

3

Therapeutic Decisions

The activities of daily living, work, and recreation provide many opportunities for protective muscle spasm to occur. Protective muscle spasm or guarding (muscle hypertonicity that occurs as the result of an injury, such as a strain; in response to abnormal biomechanics; or as a reaction to emotional stress or a pathologic process, such as inflammation) may occur with a single sudden gross movement, through repetitive smaller movements, or as a consequence of bruising, straining, or tearing.[1] Events that can result in muscle guarding include falls, catching oneself while falling, improper lifting, motor vehicle accidents, throwing injuries, and unexpected sudden movements. Most people experience several injuries over a lifetime. The injuries may be cumulative, especially if not properly treated. For example, most infants fall several times while learning how to walk. Children fall off tricycles, slides, and swings and usually experience some rough-and-tumble play. As they grow older they participate in a variety of sports and other rigorous activities. Adolescents and adults enter the workforce, and their employment may require awkward positions that involve lifting. Add to these common experiences any number of severe injuries, such as falls and motor vehicle accidents, and one can easily understand the presence of the numerous lesions that are observed clinically.

It is evident that our lives provide many opportunities for soft tissue injury to occur. The human body has an incredible ability to adapt to several minor stresses, but as soon as the number increases above a certain range, which may be different for each individual, the body has less room to adapt. Finally, it reaches a point where it cannot adapt any further. Once the physiologic adaptive range has been exceeded, there is a greater susceptibility to injury.[5] For example, a person may bend over to pick up something, an action the person has performed repeatedly without any problem. Today, however, the person's back "goes out." The injury is usually not caused by that particular movement but the accumulated stresses to the body over a lifetime. This was the "straw that broke the camel's back."

Over the years the body may develop certain areas of muscle guarding, joint hypomobility and fascial tension. This affects functional mobility and flexibility and can lead to faulty posture. When this dysfunctional body is put into motion, such as in recreational or work-related activities, or is subject to an accident, the preexisting dysfunction influences the resulting condition of the body. For example, five people involved in the same car accident may suffer completely different injuries. One may get low back pain, one may experience shoulder pain, another may get cervical and temporomandibular joint (TMJ) pain. The fourth person may feel pain in all these areas and the fifth person may not experience any pain or dysfunction. The extent of the current injury relates to the condition of the tissues at the time of the accident and the dysfunctions that were previously present. The aim of positional release therapy (PRT) is to identify areas of dysfunction and normalize the somatic tissues to improve the general condition and adability of the body.

¶WHAT IS POSITIONAL RELEASE THERAPY?

Positional release therapy is a method of total body evaluation and treatment using tender points (TPs) and a position of comfort (POC) to resolve the associated dysfunction. PRT is an *indirect* (the body part moves away from the resistance barrier, i.e., the direction of greatest ease) and *passive* (the therapist performs all the movements without help from the patient) method of treatment. All three planes of movement are used to attain the position of greatest comfort. Once the most severe tender points are found, they are palpated as a guide to help find the POC. The POC produces optimal relaxation of the involved tissues.

One theory holds that while in the position of comfort, there is a reduction and arrest of inappropriate proprioceptive activity.[6] As a result of treatment using PRT, there is a decrease in muscle tension, fascial tension, and joint hypomobility. These changes in turn result in a significant increase in functional range of motion and a decrease in pain.

¶THE EFFECTS OF POSITIONAL RELEASE THERAPY

The following are six treatment outcomes using PRT:
1. **Normalization of muscle hypertonicity.** Clinically it has been found that the first, or neuromuscular, phase of the PRT treatment lasts approximately 90 seconds for general orthopedic patients[6] and 3 minutes for neurologic patients.[13] Positional release therapy appears to affect inappropriate proprioceptive activity during this phase, thus helping to normalize tone and set the normal length-tension relationship in the muscle. This results in the elongation of the involved muscle fibers to their normal state.[6,13]
2. **Normalization of fascial tension.** It is hypothesized by D'Ambrogio[4] and Weiselfish[12,13] that the second, or fascial, phase of the PRT treatment begins after 90 seconds for general orthopedic patients and after 3 minutes for neurologic patients. During this phase, PRT apparently begins to engage the fascial tension patterns associated with trauma, inflammation, and adhesive pathology.[2,7] This process may involve an "unwinding" action in the myofascial tissue.[11] A significant release response may be palpated during this phase.
3. **Reduction of joint hypomobility.** When the muscles crossing joints become hypertonic or tight, the result is joint hypomobility (i.e., joint stiffness). By using PRT, the affected muscles and fascial tissues relax.

This appears to ease the tension around the joint, which allows it to move more freely. Therefore proper biomechanical movement is restored to the joint.
4. **Increased circulation and reduced swelling.** As the musculoskeletal structures are relaxed using PRT, pressure appears to be relieved on intervening structures such as blood and lymph vessels. The result may be increased circulation, which in turn aids in the healing of damaged tissue. The improved lymphatic drainage assists in the reabsorption of tissue fluids, thus reducing the swelling associated with inflammation.
5. **Decreased pain.** The pain of joint dysfunction is position oriented, from severe pain in one position to almost complete comfort in the opposite position. The patient has pain, which may be associated with muscle guarding, fascial tension, and restriction of joint movement. Positional release therapy appears to alleviate muscle spasm and restore proper pain-free movement and tissue flexibility. The patient may have some remaining discomfort because of residual inflammation, but the sharp pain is often significantly reduced.
6. **Increased strength.** By normalizing the proprioceptive and neural balance within muscle tissue and removing inhibition caused by pain, PRT can help restore normal tone and function of the involved muscles. Thus PRT may optimize the biomechanical efficiency of muscle and improve the responsiveness to prescribed conditioning exercises.

¶CONTRAINDICATIONS TO THE USE OF POSITIONAL RELEASE THERAPY

If the therapist is following the PRT general rules and principles as stated in Chapter 4, there are only a few contraindications to be aware of, such as malignancy, aneurysm, and acute rheumatoid arthritis. The following are regional contraindications to the use of PRT:
- Open wounds
- Sutures
- Healing fractures
- Hematoma
- Hypersensitivity of the skin
- Systemic or localized infection

The patient should always complete a thorough history and evaluation before beginning treatment. A complete diagnostic workup may also be necessary. Although a certain PRT technique may not be recommended for one area of the body because of one of the aforementioned contraindications, it may be safe to use on other regions. Always proceed with caution, taking into account the emotional state of the patient. Allow the patient to make informed decisions.[2]

When placing the patient into the position of comfort, it is imperative that the tissues be allowed to relax. There should be no palpable tenderness or pain, and the patient should never be forced into a position. It must be a comfortable process with the patient in a completely relaxed position. Although it is emphasized that the patient should experience no pain while being placed in the POC, pain or paresthesia may develop *during* the treatment. This is normal and usually lasts 1 to 2 minutes. It is part of the release process.[10,11]

Problems tend to arise when the therapist tries to force a patient into a POC. If the patient is in immediate discomfort on being placed in the position, this may indicate the presence of a conflicting lesion. In this case the therapist should search for another significant tender point or use another modality.

Special care must be taken when working on the neck with regard to the vertebral artery.[9] When extending the patient's head and neck over the end of the table, it is essential to go down the kinetic chain extremely gently, keeping the suboccipital region in flexion and axial extension. The patient's eyes must be kept open, and the therapist should monitor for signs of vertebral artery compression (such as nystagmus).[9] It is recommended that the therapist keep talking to the patient or questioning the patient regarding dizziness. It is important to use sound judgment and to ensure that the patient is always taken into a position of ease. The therapist should feel the tissues becoming relaxed. As long as these guidelines are followed, the risk of harm to the patient will be minimized.

❡Which Conditions Respond Best to Positional Release Therapy?

As mentioned earlier, PRT treats protective muscle spasm, fascial tension, and joint hypomobility, which are usually the result of a physical injury. Therefore any patient who has a distinct, physical mechanism of injury will respond favorably to PRT. These include injuries resulting from falls; improper lifting; throwing; motor vehicle accidents; sudden, unexpected movements; and sports. The degree to which the patient responds depends on the degree of dysfunction that preceded the acute injury.

Those patients whose pain commenced insidiously with no obvious immediate mechanism of injury but who have a history of trauma also tend to respond well to PRT. In these cases, the pain may be the result of surpassing a physiologic adaptive range. So-called repetitive strain injuries (RSIs) may result from excessive challenge to the acccumulated muscular guarding, fascial tension, and/or joint restrictions. Treatment directed to these background dysfunctions may allow for resolution of these types of conditions. Those patients who have had acute or chronic pain that arose insidiously with no clear mechanism of injury or history of trauma tend not to respond as well. Their dysfunctions tend to be related to stress, visceral dysfunction, pathology (e.g., infections, tumours), or surgical intervention. Initial evaluation of the patient and subjective findings should help identify these red flags. An appropriate referral for further investigation may be necessary to ascertain underlying conditions.

❡When Is It Appropriate to Use Positional Release Therapy?

There are four phases of treatment, which comprise structural and functional rehabilitation.

Phase I. This phase deals with treating patients in the acute phase of the injury. Positional release therapy is the treatment of choice in this phase and can be used immediately after injury because of its gentleness. Positional release therapy helps reset the inappropriate proprioceptive activity and decreases the amount of muscle spasm, joint hypomobility, and fascial tension. It can create a better environment for healing to take place and help decrease the sharp pain and swelling that may develop. Positional release therapy can be extremely effective in this phase of recovery and may significantly reduce downtime for athletes and help promote a rapid return to preinjury status. Once in the clinic, the therapist can also integrate other modalities, such as ice, microcurrent, pulsed ultrasound, and taping, and use of assistive devices such as canes, crutches, and splints.

Phase II. This phase deals with treating structural dysfunction with both acute and chronic patients. With chronic patients, there are usually several areas of long-standing dysfunction. Positional release therapy by itself or in conjunction with other manual therapies can be used to reduce spasm, joint hypomobility, and fascial tension. This can result in improved postural alignment and an increase in functional mobility and flexibility in the spine, ribs, pelvis, and peripheral joints. There is usually a decrease in pain. This enables the patient to move much more easily and comfortably. At this point, mobility and strengthening exercises can be added to further facilitate change and to progress the patient to the next phase. This phase prepares the patient's body for movement.

Phase III. Phase III deals with the restoration of functional movement. Once the patient has overcome the acute and structural phase, he should be moving more easily with less discomfort and be ready to progress to a more dynamic movement program. This includes cardiovascular fitness (aerobics), strengthening (weight lifting), and a continuation of flexibility and mobility exercises from phase II. The patient at this stage should not be experiencing any sharp pain, although dull pain may occur with the healing process. The patient's range of motion should be relatively pain free. The focus of therapy is on improving functional movement, strengthening muscles for structural support, and improving cardiovascular fitness.

Phase IV. Phase IV deals with normalization of life activities. It takes into consideration the patient's lifestyle and goals. Is the patient able to continue with his work, activities of daily living, and sports or recreational activities? Does he need retraining, lifestyle modification, or additional therapy? Appropriate referrals to other professionals or functional capacity evaluation should be considered to facilitate this final transitional phase.

All four phases are important, and sometimes patients must progress through all phases. However, each patient must be evaluated as an individual. For example, a patient may need only the wellness program because she is deconditioned. Another patient might require only some manual therapy. Problems can arise, for example, when a patient who has low back pain is treated only as an acute patient in phase I. The patient may be treated with ultrasound, ice, or electrical stimulation for 3 months, and then when there is no improvement, she is thrown into a work-hardening program or functional capacity evaluation. She will likely fail miserably because she is not conditioned and no one has worked on the dysfunction in her spine or peripheral joint. In some clinics, patients are put into a wellness program immediately, without any manual therapy being done. Patients must be prepared for exercises. Do they have some spinal impairment? Is there some muscle guarding, fascial tension, or joint restriction which might impede them from exercising properly? Other clinics may treat a patient with only manual therapy and without including any exercise. Consequently, it is a passive process, and the patient has no responsibilities. This approach may also fail with many patients because their dysfunction might be directly caused by a sedentary lifestyle, which has not been addressed.

To achieve success, it is essential that all patients be evaluated to determine their specific requirements. Some patients may require acute attention, such as icing or other modalities. One patient may require minimal hands-on treatment, whereas another may need extensive hands-on therapy to alleviate restricted joints, fascial restrictions, or protective muscle spasm. After treatment the patient should progress into a wellness program where his muscles are being worked appropriately, and the therapist should encourage him to exercise on his own. Finally, whether the patient can return to his previous employment must be considered. Each patient must be individually evaluated and a unique and specialized plan followed.

❚Who Can Benefit from Positional Release Therapy?

A wide assortment of patients, from infants to geriatric patients, can benefit from PRT. The human frame may be viewed as an evolutionary compromise. The bipedal posture and the wide range of motion afforded the upper limbs have allowed humans to dominate their environment. These adaptations, however, have not been without a cost. A higher center of gravity and reduced stability in the upper quadrant cause humans to be more vulnerable to translational forces and resultant musculoskeletal injuries. Positional release therapy, because of its efficiency and gentleness, is appropriate for a wide range of injuries to which humans are subject.

Treatment is always directed to the individual and the individual's unique set of dysfunctions as opposed to a diagnosed condition or group of symptoms.

CONDITIONS OF THE SPINE, RIBS, PELVIS, AND SACRUM

Patients with a herniated disk, facet impingement, stenosis, fusion, spondylolisthesis, degenerative disk disease, arthritis, scoliosis, fracture, postsurgical laminectomy, postsurgical diskectomy, Harrington rods, sacroiliac pain, lumbosacral pain, lumbar strain, myofascial pain, or coccydynia have all benefitted from PRT alone or in conjunction with other modalities. Positional release therapy is not contraindicated in patients with osteoporosis, as treatment is completely nontraumatic. As stated previously we feel that PRT does not repair these patholgic or surgical conditions. Positional Release Therapy treats the dysfunction by decreasing muscle hypertonicity, reducing fascial tension, and restoring joint mobility. As a result, the patient will begin to move more easily and with less pain. In cases of severe restriction of motion, it is possible to apply PRT only within this limited available range. The positioning will gradually approach the optimal POC; however, this may require several successive treatments. With the incorporation of mobility, flexibility, strengthening, and cardiovascular exercises, the patient should respond well.

Orthopedic surgery does not address the underlying dysfunction. There may be a postsurgical reduction in symptoms; however, this is not always the case, and relief is often of only short duration.[3] In these cases it is appropriate to treat the dysfunctions using conservative manual methods and other modalities to normalize the tissues and restore optimal biomechanics.

It is our opinion that in many cases attributed to disk pathology, arthritis, or stenosis, the symptoms may, in fact, be caused by soft tissue dysfunction. What appears as a pathology on an x-ray may be the end result of abnormal biomechanics, which is the result of the dysfunction.[8] Unfortunately, soft tissue or articular dysfunction cannot be visualized using current imaging technology, and thus the patient's symptoms are often atributed to abnormalities associated with an osseous image. Conservative functional therapies, such as PRT, should be considered before surgical options are initiated.

CONDITIONS OF THE UPPER QUADRANT

Patients who have been diagnosed with bursitis, rotator cuff tendinitis, impingement syndrome, thoracic outlet syndrome, acromioclavicular sprain, sternoclavicular sprain, postfracture conditions, frozen shoulder, tennis elbow, and golfer's elbow have benefited from PRT.

The shoulder is an inherently unstable joint and relies heavily on the muscles that cross it for support. Careful examination of all of these tissues should be carried out when locally assessing this joint. The upper limb is directly linked to the cervicothoracic spine and rib cage in relation to nerve supply, circulatory supply, and muscular and fascial extensions. It has been found clinically that disorders of the shoulder, elbow, wrist, and hand may often arise from primary dysfunctions of the axial skeleton. Commonly, significant tender points are present in the cervical spine, thoracic spine, or rib cage, that, when treated according to the general rules, help resolve many of the conditions that cause primary symptoms in the upper limb.

CONDITIONS OF THE LOWER QUADRANT

Patients with hip bursitis, tendinitis, total hip replacement, arthritis, jumper's knee, total knee replacement, patellar tendinitis, chondromalacia, meniscus tears, ligament sprain, capsulitis, and plantar fasciitis have all responded successfully to PRT. Positional release therapy addresses the functional component as opposed to the pathology. In cases of total hip and knee replacements, the tissues will still be able to guide the therapist. Sometimes the therapist may feel that the hips are being placed in a compromising position, but if the tension in the tissues is relaxing, the tenderness is disappearing, and the patient states that it feels good, she should continue with the treatment. Therefore it is important for the therapist to continually monitor for changes. Muscle guarding, strains, and sprains are common in the lower quadrant. Positional release therapy can be effective at treating injuries involving the hip, knee, ankle, and foot and can help the patient progress to a weight-bearing and walking stage quickly.

MOTOR VEHICLE ACCIDENT CASES

Patients who have been involved in a motor vehicle accident respond well to PRT, as in other cases where there is a clear mechanism of injury that is traumatic in nature. If the accident is severe and there are many conflicting tender points, a severe tender point in another area, as determined by the scanning evaluation (SE) (see Chapter 5), may need to be treated initially. Otherwise craniosacral therapy, myofascial release, or other modalities may be used as initial interventions. Once the conflicting protective muscle spasm has diminished, PRT in the local area may be instituted. If the injury is minor to moderate and it is possible to localize a distinct tender point and find a POC, the results with PRT will be good. Positional release therapy alone has helped with cervical sprains and strains, headaches, tinnitus, dizziness, and TMJ dysfunctions. Therefore, depending on the severity of the accident and which systems have been affected in the patient's body, an integration of the various manual therapies is usually effective. Early post-injury intervention has been clinically found to reduce the incidence of secondary compensations and conflicting tender points. This can simplify treatment and speed recovery.

GERIATRIC PATIENTS

Arthritic conditions may develop in one hip or knee because of biomechanical imbalances arising from previous injuries. Most elderly patients feel that the pain in their hip or knee is due to arthritis or is a factor of age. They do not believe that much can be done for them. When confronted with this argument, the therapist may wish to say to the patient, "Your right and left knees are the same age, so why did only one knee develop the arthritis?" This type of reasoning may encourage them to reconsider their limiting beliefs and thus allow them to cooperate more fully with the treatment program.

Usually, when elderly patients are exposed to PRT, they quickly accept it because it is gentle and effective. Positional release therapy may be able to release several chronic dysfunctions that have been preventing the patient from achieving a normal functional range of motion. These patients are often surprised and excited with the results. They find themselves moving more easily with less discomfort and performing movements that they have not done in years and assumed they had lost forever. These may include tying shoes, looking both ways when driving, riding a bike, walking, swimming, and other activities of daily living. Osteoporosis is a consideration with this patient population. PRT may be the treatment of choice in these cases and it is a gentle technique which the elderly generally tolerate very well.

PEDIATRIC PATIENTS

Infants and young children with torticollis, brachial plexus injuries (Erb's or mixed palsy), and colicky babies have been treated successfully with PRT. Sometimes it may be difficult to communicate effectively with this patient population, and there is a need to rely on observation and palpation skills. For example, in the case of an infant with a right-sided torticollis (i.e., right side bent and left rotated cervical spine), evaluation of the movement restrictions may reveal reduced left lateral flexion and right rotation. One may also palpate hypertonicity in the sternocleidomastoid (SCM) muscle on the right side. Treatment is a simple matter of reproducing the action of the SCM muscle. The child's neck is treated by placing the child into flexion, right lateral flexion, and left rotation. The therapist feels for softening of the involved SCM muscle as a guide. Clinically, this technique is much more effective than stretching the muscle. The child will likely be more cooperative because the treatment is more comfortable than stretching.

Infants and very young children are best treated close to their nap time or after feeding. The assessment may be performed during the initial visit without treatment, in order to gain the child's confidence. This also provides an opportunity to make the treatment session as short and efficient as possible and to arrange it at an optimal time within the child's schedule.

SPORTS INJURIES

Patients with sports injuries respond extremely well to PRT. As mentioned previously, PRT works best when there is a clearcut mechanism of injury that is traumatic in nature. With the exception of the weekend athlete, this population is in good shape and responds quickly to PRT. The younger athletes who have fewer accumulated dysfunctions respond especially well. Weekend athletes will also respond, but if they have an accumulation of dysfunctions, they may not respond as quickly.

For the most part, the treatments for this population are straightforward. Common injuries such as sprained ankles, hamstring or calf strains, knee ligament sprains, pelvic or sacroiliac strains, and rotator cuff and elbow injuries can be treated effectively using PRT in conjunction with range-of-motion exercises, strengthening exercises, and other modalities.

RESPIRATORY PATIENTS

Patients who have difficulty breathing can benefit from PRT. Many respiratory patients are taught breathing exercises for energy conservation and to improve their respiratory potential. These are functional in nature. However, restricted ribs, spine, pelvis, and hypertonic muscles may prevent these patients from achieving full functional benefit. They can only achieve a certain potential with these breathing exercises. Therefore by treating the restrictions in the spine, pelvis, ribs, and hypertonic muscles (i.e., diaphragm, psoas, quadratus lumborum, and intercostal muscles) the patient may be able to expand the rib cage more fully and with greater ease and may be able to perform breathing exercises to a greater potential and with more comfort. It is important to understand that PRT does not treat the respiratory disease but rather improves breathing mechanics, which may support the healing process, and makes the patient feel more comfortable.

AMPUTEES

Some amputees with a history of trauma (e.g., car accident) benefit from PRT. When the pelvis, sacrum, spine, and non-affected leg are treated, this may result in better alignment and comfort when sitting in a wheelchair. When the patient has pain or excessive pressure on the stump, therapists often assume that the prosthetic device needs adjusting. The practitioner should first evaluate for dysfunctions in the patient's pelvis, sacrum, spine, and other sites and provide appropriate treatment. Often, this is enough to realign the patient's body, decrease the pain, and reduce the excessive pressure or discomfort that the patient is experiencing. If pain or discomfort prevents these patients from exercising or walking, PRT can be used in conjunction with other techniques such as mat exercises, and gait and balance training.

NEUROLOGIC PATIENTS

Positional release therapy has been used successfully along with craniosacral therapy, muscle energy, and myofascial release when treating individuals with hypertonicity secondary to both upper and lower motor neuron lesions. These patients include those with traumatic brain injury, cerebral vascular accident, multiple sclerosis, cerebral palsy, and spinal cord injuries. Patients with hypotonia or atonia (i.e., flaccid arm and leg tone) are not appropriate for treatment using PRT. This is a regional consideration only; an individual may have flaccid patterns in one area of the body and a spastic pattern in another region. The hypertonic or spastic region would be amenable to treatment using PRT.

Positional release therapy may be used to normalize tone in order to assist with trunk elongation, improve pelvic positioning, and increase mobility and functional movement. Positonal release therapy helps create an improved neuromusculoskeletal environment that allows for optimal implementation of a neurodevelopmental program.

It may be difficult to communicate with this patient population. Therefore it is essential to be aware of postural dysfunction and movement restriction patterns and be able to palpate changes in tone of the affected muscles. As an example, a neurologic patient has increased flexor tone in the hips. Palpation of the involved muscles and an evaluation of the range of motion confirms this finding. This patient will tolerate flexion and external rotation of the hips but may not tolerate extension. Treatment using PRT would involve hip flexion and external rotation. The therapist would follow the ease of movement of the tissues and palpate the hip flexors to be guided into the POC. Remember that neurologic patients require an initial positioning of a minimum of 3 minutes for the neuromuscular release. A fascial release will occur after this.

For additional information regarding the treatment of the neurologic patient, refer to the list of common tender points for the neurologic patient and Weiselfish's postural pathokinesiologic model in the Appendix.

¶SUMMARY

Positional release therapy has been found clinically to work best where there has been a clear mechanism of injury, either acute or chronic in nature. Therefore history of trauma is important in the patient's initial evaluation. Positional release therapy has been found to benefit a wide assortment of patients. Positional release therapy is primarily used in the first two phases of rehabilitation, the acute and structural phases. It must be understood that PRT does not change pathologic or surgical conditions. The therapist is not treating a "diagnosis." He is treating a human being with dysfunctions. The aim of PRT is to remove restrictive barriers of movement in the body. This is accomplished by decreasing protective muscle spasm, fascial tension, joint hypomobility, pain, and swelling and increasing circulation and strength. As a result the patient begins to move more easily, with less pain and discomfort. She can then be progressed to phases III and IV, the wellness and work reconditioning phases of rehabilitation.

References

1. Anderson DL: *Muscle pain relief in 90 seconds: the fold and hold method*, Minneapolis, 1995, Chronimed.
2. Barnes J: *Myofascial release: the search for excellence*, 1990, self-published.
3. Brown CW: The natural history of thoracic disc degeneration, *Spine*, (suppl) June 1992.
4. D'Ambrogio K: *Strain/counterstrain* (course syllabus), Palm Beach Gardens, 1992, Upledger Institute.
5. Gelb H: *Killing pain without prescription*, New York, 1980, Harper & Row.
6. Jones LH: *Strain and counterstrain*, Newark, Ohio, 1981, American Academy of Osteopathy.
7. Levin SM: The icosohedron as the three-dimensional finite element in biomechanical support. Proceedings of the Society of General Systems Research on Mental Images, Valves and Reality, Philadelphia, Society of General Systems Research, May 1986.
8. Rosomoff HL and others: Physical findings in patients with chronic intractable benign pain of the neck and/or back, *Pain*, 37:279, 1989.
9. Saunders HD: *Evaluation, treatment and prevention of musculoskelatal disorders*, Minneapolis, 1989, Viking Press.
10. Smith FF: *Inner bridges—a guide to energy movement and body structure*, Atlanta, 1986, Humanics New Age.
11. Upledger JE: *Crainiosacral therapy*, Seattle, 1983, Eastland Press.
12. Weiselfish S: *Manual therapy for the orthopedic and neurologic patient emphasizing strain and counterstrain technique*, Hartford, Conn, 1993, Regional Physical Therapy, self-published.
13. Weiselfish S: Personal communication, 1995.

4

Clinical Principles

This chapter outlines the clinical significance of the tender point (TP), identifies where to find TPs, and explains how to grade the severity of their tenderness. It explains how to prioritize these tender points in order to prepare a treatment plan and explains the general rules and principles to follow when performing positional release therapy (PRT). The frequency, duration, and scheduling of treatments are discussed. It is important to understand the general principles so that the treatment sessions will be as efficient as possible.

Before beginning treatment, it is important to understand the difference between *global* and *local* treatment. The scanning evaluation (SE) will reveal the most clinically significant lesions. There may be several significant lesions as the result of successive injuries, creating a layering effect of the dysfunction pattern. This pattern of interrelated lesions is referred to as the *global dysfunction.*

Given the presence of several possible significant lesions within the global dysfunction, the practitioner must nevertheless find a place to begin therapy. By comparing these lesions in a sequential manner, the practitioner will be able to determine the one or two dominant lesions, each of which is represented by a dominant tender point (DTP). The primary aim of therapy is to treat the global dysfunction via the DTPs because this pattern represents the source of the patient's symptoms.

For example, in Fig. 4-1 a patient develops symptoms in his right knee as a result of running. The patient has a hypomobile right S-I joint that is causing excessive pronation in the right foot and ankle. If there is prolonged pronation during toe off this will result in internal rotation of the tibia and external rotation of the femur, causing a torque through the knee Over time this can lead to the development of symptoms in the right knee. If one were to treat only the symptoms the problem would persist. Treating globally first (i.e., the hypmobile right S-I joint) would reduce the torque on the knee and reduce the chance of reoccurrence. After treating the global dysfunction, the therapist may elect to treat the knee locally for symptomatic relief.

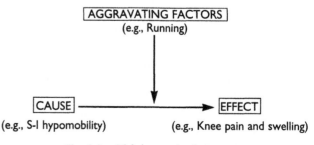

Fig. 4-1 *Global versus local treatment.*

¶WHAT IS THE CLINICAL SIGNIFICANCE OF THE TENDER POINT?

A tender point may be defined as a tense, tender, edematous region that is located deep in muscles, tendons, ligaments, fascia, or bone. It can measure 1 cm across or less, with the most acute point being about 3 mm in diameter. Tension is also felt in the tissues surrounding the tenderness. The tender point is usually four times as sensitive as normal tissue.[5] As mentioned in Chapters 1 and 2, the tender points associated with PRT share common characteristics and locations with trigger points,[8] neurolymphatic points,[3] neurovascular points,[1,2] and acupuncture (Ah Shi points).[6] Most people feel that the tender point itself is the dysfunction. However, it is only an outward manifestation of the reaction of the tissues to an underlying lesion. Patients often find it interesting to learn that there is tenderness in a body region that is not obviously painful for them. They often have no palpable tenderness in the area of pain.

¶WHERE ARE THE TENDER POINTS?

Tender points are found throughout the body, anteriorly, posteriorly, medially, and laterally. A diagram of these tender points is shown in the Appendix. As illustrated, these tender points are found on muscle origins or insertions, within the muscle belly, over the ligaments, tendons, fascia, and bone.

¶HOW HARD SHOULD TENDER POINTS BE PALPATED DURING THE ASSESSMENT?

When documenting the tender points, the tissue should not be pressed so hard that tenderness on all the points is elicited. Likewise, if the touch is too light tender points may be missed. There is no substitute for clinical experience and objective trial and error. We recommend that the practitioner find one tender point on the patient and then determine how little pressure is required to elicit the *jump sign*. A jump sign is characterized by certain responses, such as a sudden jerking motion, grabbing of the therapist's hand, a facial grimace, or the expression of a vocal expletive. Through practice, the precise degree of pressure will be learned. The depth of the tissue being palpated must also be considered. Deeper tissue requires more pressure than superficial tissue, but it must be done gently and with finesse. It is important to be firm when palpating, but tissue must be entered gently, and only necessary pressure must be used to palpate through the layers of tissue. The patient being evaluated should be taken into account. Babies, children, athletes, and elderly patients may respond differently to touch. Patients' belief systems, how much pain they are in, and how frail their bodies are can all be factors in determining the amount of pressure that may be used to palpate.

● - Extremely sensitive

◖ - Very sensitive

◗ - Moderately sensitive

○ - No tenderness

Fig. 4-2 *System used to grade the severity of tender points.*

¶HOW IS THE SEVERITY OF TENDERNESS GRADED?

When evaluating the body for tender points, a grading system is necessary in order to measure the severity of each point. In this text, four circles with various amounts of shading as shown in Fig. 4-2 are used to grade the severity of the tender points.

When palpating a patient who has an extremely sensitive tender point, there is a visual jump sign, and the patient will express extreme sensitivity to touch. This point is labeled *extremely sensitive*, and in the SE the entire circle is shaded (●). If the point is very tender but there is no jump sign, the point is labeled *very sensitive* and only the top half of the circle is filled in (◖). The patient states that the point is very tender but does not flinch or jump away when TP is touched.

If the patient notices some tenderness of the point but there is no jump sign, it is labeled *moderate* and only the bottom half of the circle is filled in (◗). If there is *no tenderness* at all, the circle is left blank (○). The Scanning Evaluation Recording Sheet is shown in the Appendix.

¶WHAT HAPPENS IF THE PATIENT IS UNABLE TO COMMUNICATE?

The inability to directly communicate the severity of tenderness is a factor with certain neurologic patients and infants, among others. Occasionally a jump sign may be detected with palpation. If not, other cues must be used. Posture, range of motion, and tension in the muscle must be evaluated and used as a guide. Weiselfish has developed a chart to evaluate movement and postural restrictions associated with tender points to assist therapists treating these types of patients. (See p. 243 in the Appendix for an example of the postural pathokinesiologic model[10] for determination of treatment.) For example, if a patient has a right protracted shoulder, she might be able to horizontally adduct with ease but find difficulty with horizontal abduction. Tension may also be found on palpation of the right pectoralis minor. In this situation, hypertonicity of the right pectoralis minor would be indicated based on observation of the patient's posture, evaluation of movement restrictions, and palpation of tension within the muscle belly itself.

Some neurologic patients who have significant hip flexor tone are able to flex their hips with ease but find great difficulty extending their hips. Common points for these patients would be the iliacus point or the medial hamstring point. This technique may be used throughout the body.

Weiselfish, who specializes in the treatment of neurologic patients, has compiled a list of common PRT points for neurologic patients for both the upper and lower quadrants. These are found on p. 242 in the Appendix.

¶PREPARING A POSITIONAL RELEASE THERAPY TREATMENT PLAN

Before preparing a treatment plan, the body must be scanned for tender points. The Appendix contains an example of the Scanning Evaluation and Tender Point Body Chart. Once all these points have been recorded, the general rules and principles are used to prioritize the TPs and to ultimately determine the DTP, which will be treated first. These general rules and principles were developed by Dr. Jones from over 40 years of clinical experience. By following these guidelines, treatments will be much more effective and efficient.

The most important rule is to *treat the most severe tender point first.* The second most important rule is *treat proximal to distal.*[5] The second rule is required if there are equally sensitive tender points proximally and distally. For example, if there is a tender point in the neck and the shoulder, and they are equally sensitive, the neck is treated first. If it is found that the shoulder is more sensitive, the proximal/distal rule is superceded by the first rule, which is to treat the most severe tender point first.

A third type of situation can arise. If there are several areas of extremely sensitive tender points, treat the area with the greatest number of TP's first. If several equally sensitive tender points are found in a row (for example, on the anterior aspect of the sternum, i.e., if the anterior first to anterior seventh points are all equally tender), the one in the middle is treated first. This will be the point that is monitored for this group of tender points. If there are only two points, side by side, and they are equally tender, they can be monitored together. The key is to pick one point in the middle to represent the rest of the group, and in general it will be found that they will all shut off with the same treatment position.[4,5] Based on this hierarchy, the therapist should be able to identify one or more DTPs, which will be the focus of treatment.

General Rules for Preparing a PRT Treatment Plan:
1. Treat the most severe tender point first.
2. Treat the more proximal or medial tender points before those that are more distal or lateral.
3. Treat the area of greatest accumulation of tender points first.
4. When tender points are in a row, treat the one near the middle of the row first.

¶GENERAL PRINCIPLES OF TREATMENT

Jones's general treatment procedure was basically to fold the body part over the tender point to shorten and relax the affected muscles and other soft tissues. This has been found to be a useful guide in many cases. However, there are some exceptions, and these are identified in Chapter 6. Following are four basic rules developed by Jones that should be observed when attempting to treat a tender point.
1. Anterior tender points are usually treated in flexion. For example, see the treatment position for IL on p. 151 of Chapter 6.
2. Posterior tender points are treated in extension. For example, see the treatment position for PL3 on p. 162 of Chapter 6.
3. If a tender point is on or near the midline, it is treated with more pure flexion for anterior points and with more pure extension for posterior points. For example, see treatment position AT1 → AT6 on p. 86 (Chapter 6) and the treatment position of UPL5 on p. 164 of Chapter 6.
4. If the tender point is lateral to the midline, it is treated with the addition of side bending, rotation, or both. The anterior/flexion or posterior/extension rule must also be followed. For example, see the treatment position AR3-10 on p. 93 of Chapter 6.[5]

¶WHAT IS THE COMFORT ZONE?

A key concept to understand is that PRT is an indirect technique, meaning the body is taken into a position of ease away from the resistance barrier. For example, if the patient has hypertonicity of the long head of the biceps, the patient will feel tension in that muscle if the elbow is extended. The patient will find it more comfortable to flex the elbow, causing shortening of the biceps, whereas extension would challenge the resistance in the affected muscle. Therefore in PRT the painful and restricted position is avoided, and the goal is to find a position of ease. The optimal position of ease is the *comfort zone* (CZ). Figure 4-3 illustrates the relationship of the CZ to the position of the body and the method used to find the comfort zone for the long head of the biceps. The vertical axis represents the severity of tenderness and palpable tissue tension or tone for the long head of the biceps tender point. The scale ranges from 0 to 10, with 0 representing complete comfort with no tenderness and minimal tissue tension and 10 representing extreme tenderness and maximal palpable tissue tension. The horizontal axis represents the range of motion of the elbow from 0° to 150° of elbow flexion. It is apparent that large movements from 0° to 110° of flexion produce little change in the tenderness level. However, with movement from 115° to 120°, which is only a 5° range, there is a dramatic change in the tenderness/tension level. A position is then reached at which there is no tenderness and the tissues are completely relaxed; this is the comfort zone. Moving to

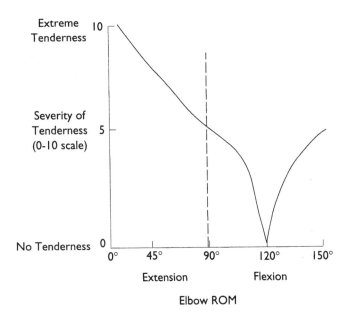

Fig. 4-3   *Comfort zone of the long head of the biceps. (Modified from Jones LH: Strain and counterstrain, Newark, Ohio, 1981, American Academy of Osteopathy.)*

the left of the CZ on the diagram, into extension, will induce increased tenderness and tension in the tissues. With movement further to the right of the comfort zone, into flexion, an increase in tenderness and tension in the tissues will again be encountered. In the latter case, the response of the tissues may be the result of engaging the antagonist (for example, the triceps), placing it into relative stretch and thus creating an increase in proprioceptive stimulation that would then feed back to the agonist (biceps).[5]

¶ACHIEVING THE OPTIMAL POSITION OF COMFORT

Achieving the optimal POC is the ultimate goal of treatment and the one that requires the greatest degree of clinical finesse. This will determine the ultimate success of the therapeutic intervention. The comfort zone is specific and is different for each of the treatment positions. As the practitioner treats the patient and attempts to find the comfort zone, the use of fine movements will be necessary as the CZ is approached, in order to avoid missing the small range of motion in which it appears. The signals that indicate that the optimal CZ has been attained include a dramatic reduction in tenderness and a significant, palpable softening of the tissues in the area of the tender point. A position will be reached at which there is no tenderness and the tissue is completely softened around the palpating finger. The response of the tender point can vary from patient to patient. Some patients have easily detected comfort zones; in others the response will be more difficult to ascertain. When trying to shut off a tender point, the key is perseverance.

It is important to remember that it is essential, while moving the patient's body into the treatment position, to maintain contact with the tender point being treated. Contact is maintained by keeping a gentle touch on the tender point, *not* by applying additional pressure.[5] As the comfort zone is approached, increased pressure must be applied periodically to the tender point to monitor its progress. However, as soon as the comfort zone is reached, contact should be maintained but no additional pressure applied. It is the position in which the patient has been placed that is the treatment, not the pressure on the tender point, which is primarily a monitor to help locate this position of ease. (Chaitow[2] contends that even light pressure on the tender point may exert a therapeutic effect.) While the patient is in the POC, pressure may be added intermittently to confirm that the ideal position is being properly maintained.

An important point to note is that as the patient is being placed into the POC he should be pain free. If any pain is experienced while the patient is being positioned, it is not the correct position for him. For example, although an anterior tender point may improve by flexing the patient, a posterior tender point may be stressed, which is more significant, thus requiring primary treatment. A thorough evaluation before treatment will reduce the likelihood of this occurring. Discomfort or other sensations arising after the POC has been achieved (generally after 30 to 60 seconds) are usually a part of the normal release process and tend to subside after another 1 to 3 minutes. It has been found that having the patient take a deep breath in and out releases tension in the affected tissues. The use of either traction or compression in small amounts may also help with the complete resolution of the tender point. Once the position is close to the comfort zone, it is important to make the movements as small as possible to fine-tune the positioning.

¶HOW LONG IS THE POSITION OF COMFORT MAINTAINED?

Once the patient is in a position of comfort, the difficult phase of the treatment is over. Now it is a waiting game. According to Jones, 90 seconds is sufficient for release of tension in the muscle tissue, and this has been backed up by 30 years of clinical experience.[5] According to Weiselfish and D'Ambrogio, there are two phases to the release of the tender points. The first phase is a length-tension change in the muscle tissue itself, which takes approximately 90 seconds for routine orthopedic patients. Weiselfish has found that the change in the length-tension relationship with the muscle will take approximately 3 minutes with neurologic patients.[10] While in the POC the patient may be surprised that the point is no longer tender and will frequently ask if the therapist is still on the same point. The second phase of treatment is a fascial release component and may take anywhere from 5 to 20 minutes to resolve. Times vary from patient to patient depending on the dysfunction.

Therefore in answering the initial question, "How long do we hold a patient in the position of comfort?" the answer is "The patient's body will tell you." This approach to positional release was referred to by such pioneers as Hoover as early as the 1940s. (See Chapter 1.) While the patient is in the comfort zone, the tissues are being palpated for a *release phenomenon*.[7,9] The release phenomenon, which can be felt by both the patient and the therapist, signifies a normalization of the tissues. The therapist monitors for relaxation and softening in the tissues, pulsation, vibration, heat, and changes in perspiration. Changes in breathing rhythm, heart rate, and eye motor activity may also be detected. These responses occur during the treatment, and once these changes cease the treatment is over and the patient often experiences a deep sense of relaxation. The therapist can help the patient feel these sensations by identifying them as they occur. The patient may also experience some achiness, pain, or paresthesia. Reassure the patient that these sensations are transitory, tending to dissipate within a minute or two, and are usually followed by a further release of tension. Each patient will be different, and the patient's body will dictate how long the patient needs to be in the position of comfort. While the patient is in the POC, it is up to the practitioner to monitor for the release phenomenon. If there is pain while getting into the position of comfort, that is a contraindication for that position.

THE IMMEDIATE POSTTREATMENT RESPONSE

It is important to mention that once the point has been fully released the body must return to a neutral position *slowly* especially for the first 15° of motion. It is hypothesized that the ballistic proprioceptors will be reengaged by returning to neutral too quickly. This may result in the reestablishment of the protective muscle spasm. After returning to neutral, the tender point must be rechecked. During this entire process, the therapist's finger should remain over the tender point. This point should be either fully eliminated or at least 70% improved.[5] There should also be immediate changes in the patient's pain level, posture, muscle tension, joint mobility, and biomechanical movement. After treating this point, the other significant points noted in the screening evaluation should be rechecked. Some of the other points will be found to have been completely released or significantly reduced in severity. Then, using the general rules and principles, the practitioner should decide which is the next most severe point to be treated, and then the whole process is repeated.

After the treatment, the patient will feel a sense of relaxation in that area. She will often find that she is able to move more easily and with less discomfort.

In the next 24 to 48 hours, clinical experience has demonstrated that approximately 40% of patients feel some increased soreness. This soreness may be found not only in the region treated but also in areas remote from the treatment area. For example, if the sacrum was treated, the patient might experience some pain in his neck or shoulder for the next few days.

It is extremely important to explain to all patients that there may be some increased soreness. It may be explained as a natural part of the body's healing process and the soft tissue reorganization taking place. If the patient is not warned of the possibility of soreness, confidence in the therapist may be diminished.

FREQUENCY, DURATION, AND SCHEDULING OF TREATMENT

It is important to be thorough on the initial evaluation because this will save much time and frustration later on. If the patient has several areas of dysfunction, that is, has had surgeries, fractures, motor vehicle accidents, or pain that is chronic in nature, an evaluation without treatment is recommended during the first visit. This is both to save time and to minimize sensory overload because the examination itself may temporarily activate several of the dysfunctions. After an evaluation, a treatment plan is prepared for future sessions. If the patient does not possess multiple dysfunctions (for example, if the injury is acute or involves a specific mechanism of injury), treatment may begin immediately after evaluation. It is recommended that a thorough PRT scanning evaluation of the patient's body be performed on the initial visit.

Remember, tender points represent dysfunctions in the patient's body, and the aim is to treat dysfunction. Pain is the end result of dysfunction. If only the painful areas are examined, the treatment will not be as effective or efficient. The goal is not to treat all the patient's tender points but to use the general rules and principles to help find the most dominant point in the patient's body, treat it, and then move on to the next most dominant point.

Positional release therapy treatment differs from that described by Jones and other practitioners. With conventional counterstrain and other forms of positional release, a patient with shoulder pain is treated using the same general rules and principles. Therapy is mainly localized to that upper quadrant, and six to eight points might be treated for a total of 90 seconds each. With global PRT sessions, only one to three points are usually treated. The goal is to spend more time on evaluation and less time on treatment. If the most dominant point of the body is located and treated, a majority of the other tender points (which may be adaptations to the dominant lesion) will often be eliminated. The dominant point may be located anywhere in the body, often remote from the area of symptoms. To achieve maximal benefit, both a muscular release and a fascial release should be obtained. This can take from 5 to 10 minutes and occasionally up to 20 minutes in the position of comfort. Each patient is different, and the release phenomenon must be felt. By persisting until a complete release is achieved, much time and needless treatment will be saved because many of the secondary tender points will be eliminated. The patient may not come in for another manual therapy session for another week or longer. During that time, the patient may be seen two to three times per week for local PRT sessions, which are held for 90 seconds, exercise therapy, the application of modalities, correction of body mechanics, ergonomic education, and other forms of supportive care. The goal with PRT is to help decrease pain, muscular hypertonicity, fascial tension, and joint hypomobility and to encourage the patient to take an active role in recovery. Clinically it has been found that it is better to perform manual therapy once a week and use the other days for exercise, modalities, and education. This allows the patient's body to adapt to the changes made during the manual therapy session. It has been found clinically that approximately 40% of patients will experience a degree of soreness for a few days following the treatment. For this reason, modality and movement therapies may be beneficial during the remainder of the week following initial treatment. (This usually only occurs after the first one or two visits.) When the patient returns for the next manual therapy session in one week to ten days, a re-evaluation should be performed using the general rules and principles to find the next most dominant lesion and treat it if necessary.

In the Scanning Evaluation Recording Sheet (see p. 232) there are five circles, which represent five treatment days. These five circles represent each of the manual therapy days. If PRT has not made any significant changes in three to five visits, there may be another system involved or it may be a red flag for a fracture, dislocation, torn tissue, infection, malignancy, or emotional stress. The patient should then be reexamined. It is important to understand that PRT is not a panacea.

SUMMARY

There are nine important points to remember when performing PRT:

1. **Scan the body, grade the severity of the tender points, and record the findings.**
2. **Follow the general rules.** It is important that the therapist treat the most severe tender point first regardless of where the pain is. Remember that the tender point represents the patient's dysfunction. The aim is to treat that dysfunction. Pain is a result of dysfunction. Once the tender point is treated and movement is restored, the pain will eventually subside. The second most important rule is to treat proximal to distal. If there are two equal tender points, treat proximally before distally. This often eliminates most of the distal tender points. With several areas of extreme sensitivity, treat the area with the greatest number of TP's first. Lastly treat the tender point in the middle of a row of equally tender points. By following these simple rules, the efficiency and effectiveness of treatment will be enhanced.
3. **Monitor the tender point while finding the position of comfort.** It is important that while placing the patient into the position of comfort, the therapist

continues to monitor the tender point the entire time. It should be monitored for a decrease in tension and tenderness. This feedback is necessary in order to assist in the fine tuning required to locate the precise comfort zone.

4. **Maintain contact on the tender point while in the position of comfort.** The tender point should be monitored throughout the treatment. Attention should be given to the changes taking place in the area of the TP, such as pulsation, heat release, vibration, unwinding, and the release in the patient's body that indicates when treatment is over. Once the treatment is over, contact should be maintained to be certain that the same spot that was evaluated before treatment is being reevaluated. When patients notice that the point is no longer tender, they will often ask, "Are you sure you are on the same point?"
5. **Hold the position of comfort until a complete release is felt.** The position of comfort is held as long as necessary to obtain a complete release in the body (i.e., a sense of relaxation in the muscle, a decrease in the heat emitted, an elimination of achiness, cessation of pulsation, vibration, or unwinding taking place in the tissue, and a relaxation of the breathing). If the patient is removed from the position of comfort too soon, the results will be more short term and the tender point may reappear and require further treatment. It is important to remember that when treating globally, the POC is usually held longer (e.g., 5-10 min) and will have a more profound effect on the body. Local treatments are usually held for approximately 90 seconds.
6. **Return to neutral slowly.** It is important to mention that once a tender point has been treated successfully, the patient's body must be returned to neutral slowly. The first 15° is the most important range. If the patient is taken out of the comfort zone too quickly, the ballistic proprioceptors may then be reengaged and the protective muscle spasm can return. These tissues are often connected to a facilitated segment, which renders them more vulnerable to reinjury and to the reestablishment of inflammation and spasm. (See Chapter 2.)
7. **Recheck the tender point and use other reality checks after treatment.** After successfully treating a tender point, it is important for the therapist and the patient to note what changes have taken place. The patient may be excited that there is a significant reduction in tenderness. However, this by itself may not be enough. It is important to have several reality checks. A reality check is finding a position, movement, or specific joint, fascial, or muscle evaluation that is objective, can be measured, and will reproduce the patient's pain or complaint. For example, a low back patient might have limitation in extension and left side bending in the quarter range, which might

increase the pain to 9 out of 10. A knee patient may have limitation in knee flexion to approximately 30° with pain at 8 out of 10. A shoulder patient may have limitations of abduction to 60° and external rotation to 30° with 9 out of 10 pain rating on both at the end of the available range. After treating with PRT, it is important to recheck these movements to see if the patient is functionally moving better with less discomfort. If these changes are not demonstrable, the treatment may not have addressed a primary lesion. These tests are an important source of feedback and can help the practitioner determine the future direction of the treatment program. They are also useful in encouraging the patient and engaging her cooperation in the recovery process.

8. **Warn the patient of possible reactions and to avoid strenuous activity after treatment.** The patient who is forewarned of the possible reactions to treatment will not only cooperate with the therapy program, but will also gain an appreciation for the power of this apparently simple and painless technique. The avoidance of strenuous activity for 24 to 48 hours after treatment will help ensure a more efficient recovery and reduce unnecessary discomfort. Failure to warn the patient may result in a loss of confidence in and cooperation with the rehabilitation program.

9. **Treat only once per week, and allow the body to adapt to the treatment.** Use PRT to remove barriers to movement, which will allow the patient to progress with activities of daily living and a functional rehabilitation program.

References

1. Bennett R: In Chapman's Reflexes. In Martin R, editor: *Dynamics of correction of abnormal function*, Sierre Madre, Calif, 1977, self-published.
2. Chaitow L: *The acupuncture treatment of pain*, Wellingborough, 1976, Thorsons.
3. Chapman F, Owens C: *Introduction to and endocrine interpretation of Chapman's reflexes*, self-published.
4. D'Ambrogio K: *Strain/counterstrain* (course syllabus), Palm Beach Gardens, 1992, Upledger Institute.
5. Jones LH: *Strain and counterstrain*, Newark, Ohio, 1981, American Academy of Osteopathy.
6. O'Connor J, Bevsky D: *Acupuncture: a comprehensive text*, Seattle, 1988, Eastland Press.
7. Smith FF: *Inner bridges—a guide to energy movement and body structure*, Atlanta, 1986, Humanics New Age.
8. Travell JG, Simons DG: *Myofascial pain and dysfunction: the trigger point manual*, Baltimore, 1983, Williams & Wilkins.
9. Upledger JE: *Craniosacral therapy*, Seattle, 1983, Eastland Press.
10. Weiselfish S: *Manual therapy for the orthopedic and neurologic patient emphasizing strain and counterstrain technique*, Hartford, Conn, 1993, Regional Physical Therapy, self-published.

5

Positional Release Therapy Scanning Evaluation

The Scanning Evaluation (SE) outlined in this chapter was designed by one of us (D'Ambrogio). The SE recording sheet and tender point body charts in the Appendix are very simple to use and are cross-referenced with Chapter 6, the treatment section of this book. These can be photocopied and used to assist in the evaluation of patients.

¶ PURPOSE OF THE SCANNING EVALUATION

The purpose of the SE is to evaluate the entire body for tender points (TPs) and to prioritize them according to their severity. In this context the TPs represent musculoskeletal dysfunction. As in most other techniques, treatment is the easy part. The difficult question is, "Where does one begin treating?" The SE, if used properly, will provide a clear, visual representation of the location of the dysfunctions that are contributing to the symptoms. In Chapter 4, the term *tender point* was defined, and an explanation was given of where and how to find these points. The prioritization of the TPs using the general rules and principles was also discussed. By recording the severity of the tender points in the SE, the practitioner will have created an organized chart of the most significant tender points, which can then be specifically categorized according to their clinical significance. This information will allow the practitioner to determine the dominant

tender point (DTP), and the treatment plan can then be implemented.

The SE should be considered an assessment tool to work in conjunction with the normal battery of orthopedic and neurologic tests (range of motion, strength testing, nerve conduction, pain questionnaires, etc.). Because this book deals mainly with positional release therapy (PRT), these other evaluation methods will not be reviewed. They are already adequately covered in several other books.

If time is taken to understand and implement the SE and PRT techniques, treatments will be much more effective and efficient. Several patients may have the same complaint (e.g., knee pain, shoulder pain, or low back pain) but the source of the condition, as revealed by the SE, may be different for each. No two patients are the same, no matter how similar their presentations may be. The PRT scanning evaluation will precisely reveal the source of the dysfunction through to DTP. By identifying the location of the key dysfunctions (which may have different locations than the perceived pain) and treating restrictive muscular and fascial barriers, the pain will begin to subside. As we continue to use the SE, we may begin to reexamine our thoughts about the body, where pain originates, and how dysfunction and pain interact. Let us now look at the SE recording sheet in detail. If you turn to the Appendix you will see a full view of the SE. You can refer back to the SE as we break it down into its components and explain step by step the nuts and bolts of how to record tender points, prioritize your findings using the general rules, and prepare a treatment plan.

Positional Release Therapy Scanning Evaluation

Patient's Name _____   Practitioner _____

Dates 1 ___ 2 ___ 3 ___ 4 ___ 5 ___

○ Extremely sensitive   ○ very   ○ moderate   ○ no tenderness
\ right   / left   + most sensitive   ○ treatment

At the top of the scanning evaluation, fill in the patient's and practitioner's name. We have included five treatment dates. These five treatment dates correspond to the five circles that you see beside each of the numbers and abbreviations of the treatment names. For example, no. 40 in Chapter 6, Section IV, Anterior Thoracic Spine, looks like this:

40. AT1 ○○○○○

The five circles are used to help us evaluate the extent of the dysfunction for each area of the body. The circles should be filled in with a pen or pencil appropriately as follows:

●-Extremely sensitive   ◔-Very   ◒-Moderate   ○-No tenderness

The key is used to record the severity of the tender points. If a point is palpated and there is an observable *jump sign* (wherein the patient responds with a jerking motion, pulling away from the contact, with facial grimace or vocal expletive), label that point *extremely sensitive* and fill in the whole circle (●). If the patient feels that the point is very tender but does not have the jump sign, the point is *very tender* and the top part of the circle is filled in (◔). If the patient has no jump sign and feels only a moderate amount of tenderness, the point is *moderately sensitive* and the bottom part of the circle is filled in (◒). If the patient experiences *no tenderness* whatsoever, the point is left blank (○).

After recording the severity of the tender point by filling in the circle, its location is noted. If, for example, a central point is found on the superior aspect of the manubrium and it is extremely tender, the circle for no. 40, AT1, is marked as follows: ●. However, if a tender point is found on either side of the body (for example, no. 170, MK), the following keys are used to label it properly:

\ Right   / Left   + Most sensitive   ⊙ Treated

For example:

170. MK ● ⟋   This means that the extremely sensitive tender point is found on the medial aspect of the left knee.

170. MK ● ⟍   This means that the extremely sensitive tender point is found on the medial aspect of the right knee.

If an extremely sensitive tender point is found equally on both points, fill in the circle and do not put any lines underneath (●). If an extremely sensitive tender point is found on both sides, but the right side appears more tender, draw slashing lines to the left and the right and place a crossing line through the one on the right. If the point is extremely sensitive on the right but only moderately or very sensitive on the left, it is recorded in the same manner.

170. MK ●⤬

When a point is treated during a session, place a small dot over the filled-in circle (●̇). It is important to identify which point was treated so that the effects of those treatments can be observed during reevaluation of the patient at subsequent sessions. Finding and treating the most severe tender point often results in the elimination of many of the secondary tender points, which may have been adapting around the primary dysfunction. This procedure is what affords PRT such a high degree of efficiency and effectiveness.

There are approximately 210 points, and each point has a number, an abbreviation, and five circles to the right. During the initial evaluation, palpate the patient's body for tender points and record them on the recording sheet. Use the key given at the beginning of this section to grade the tender points. On the initial evaluation, fill in only the first circle of each number. If there is no tenderness, leave the point blank (○). In the example below, it is found that no. 40, AT1, is the most severe tender point, the recording would appear as follows:

IV. Anterior Thoracic Spine [p. 85]

40. AT1 ●○○○○   43. AT4 ◒○○○○   46. AT7 ○○○○○   50. AT10 ○○○○○
41. AT2 ◒○○○○   44. AT5 ○○○○○   47. AT8 ◔○○○○   51. AT11 ○○○○○
42. AT3 ◒○○○○   45. AT6 ○○○○○   48. AT9 ◒○○○○   52. AT12 ○○○○○

Once the therapist has identified the DTP from the SE using the general rules and principles, the position of treatment should be looked up in Chapter 6. The exact page reference is provided in the SE recording sheet in brackets to the right of the section heading that is cross referenced with Chapter 6. In this example the DTP is no. 40 AT1. If you look to the right of the heading IV Anterior Thoracic Spine you will see the page reference (p. 85). If you turn to p. 85 you will see an illustration of all the anterior thoracic tender points. If you turn the page over and look up No. 40, which is found on p. 86, you will see:

- A sketch of the involved anatomy with the TP superimposed on it
- A photograph of the location of the TP
- A description of how to find the location of the TP
- A photo of how to perform the treatment
- A description of how to position the patient in the treatment

As you can see the SE is very user friendly and will assist you in the planning and implementation of your treatments.

Therefore one can quickly appreciate the simplicity of the scanning evaluation. First use the Tender Point Body Chart showing all of the tender points as a guide. Then record the tender points on the SE recording sheet, using the keys given on p. 232 to grade the severity. Then use the general rules and principles from (Chapter 4) to prioritize the tender points. Once the tender points that require treatment have been located, refer to the page number for the corresponding treatment section (Chapter 6). In the treatment section, you will find a sketch of that particular part of the body, with the dysfunction indicated by name, a description of the location of the tender point, and the position of treatment. Any necessary clinical notes are also included. A photograph demonstrating the most common position of treatment is also provided to help visualize the correct procedure. Therefore the scanning evaluation, when combined with the treatment section of the text, provides a user-friendly road map to an effective treatment program.

HOW TO PREPARE A TREATMENT PLAN

Follow these steps to prepare a treatment plan:
1. Scan the body for TP using the TP body chart as a guide, and record your findings appropriately on the SE recording sheet using the key provided.
2. On the first visit, record the date and fill in only the first circle for each point that is tender. The other four circles are used on subsequent visits.
3. Determine the DTP using the following four general rules and principles:
    a. Treat the most severe tender point first.
    b. Treat the more proximal or medial tender points before those that are more distal or lateral.
    c. Treat the area of the greatest accumulation of tender points first.
    d. When tender points are in a row, treat the one nearest the middle of the row first.
4. Once the DTP has been found look up the position of treatment in Chapter 6 from the page reference provided in the SE recording sheet.
5. On the subsequent visit repeat steps 1 to 4 and use the second circle to record the findings. This is continued until all five circles have been used up or patient's symptoms have subsided.

For example:

IV. Anterior Thoracic [p. 85]

40. AT1 ●●○○○	43. AT4 ○○○○○	46. AT7 ●●○○○	49. AT10 ◐○○○○
41. AT2 ●○○○○	44. AT5 ○○○○○	47. AT8 ◐○○○○	50. AT11 ○○○○○
42. AT3 ◐○○○○	45. AT6 ○○○○○	48. AT9 ○○○○○	51. AT12 ●●○○○

On the first visit AT1, AT2, AT7, and AT12 were all extremely sensitive; AT3 and AT8 were very sensitive; and AT4 and AT10 were moderately sensitive. AT7 was treated during the first visit. As a result of the treatment, we are left with AT1 extremely sensitive and AT7 and AT12 very sensitive. AT1 was treated during the second visit, and, as a result, all the points were resolved.

There are a total of five circles, representing five treatment days. Normally this is sufficient to eliminate all of the tender points. The scanning evaluation will also help identify any red flags. For example, if a tender point persists in being extremely sensitive after each visit and PRT does not seem to be shutting off that point, there may be another point in the body which is also extremely sensitive that must be treated before this. There may also be a pathologic condition or visceral disorder causing this dysfunction. This is explained in greater detail in Chapter 7, which will identify different treatment strategies.

If the time is taken to do a full evaluation of the patient on the first visit, a clear picture will form showing the locations of all the dysfunctions. Then, by using the general rules and prioritizing the tender points, a treatment plan may be formulated. It is worth repeating that it is very important to *treat the most severe tender point first* no matter where the pain seems to be because a tender point represents the dysfunction. The objective is to treat dysfunctions rather than symptoms. By using the scanning evaluation to assist in pinpointing dysfunctions, the number of dysfunctions will be reduced significantly, proper functional movement will be restored, and eventually the pain will subside.

Following are two case studies to illustrate how to use the scanning evaluation.

Case Study 1

Patient: Male in his early thirties.
Diagnosis: Medial collateral ligament strain, second degree, right knee.
Mechanism of injury: Patient states that four days prior he jumped off a 5 ft. high wall, experiencing a valgus stress to his right knee before landing on his back. Patient experienced immediate pain and swelling to his right knee.
Weight-bearing status: Patient was weight bearing as tolerated with crutches and was wearing a knee immobilizer on his right knee.
Range of motion: Knee extension -8°, knee flexion 25°.
Pain: Patient was in constant pain that varied in intensity. He would always feel a baseline of soreness and stiffness at approximately 5/10 on the pain scale. This pain could increase to 10/10 if he was on his feet for a prolonged time, which meant more than one half hour, or if he made a quick rotational movement or tried to move his knee beyond its available range.
Palpation: Patient was tender in the medial aspect of the knee with some warmth and swelling evident. On specific positional release PRT evaluation, his most dominant tender point was found to be in the paraspinal muscles at L3 posteriorly (PL3). Even though there was some soreness and palpable tenderness in and around the knee, there was no comparison to the observable jump sign he had on palpation of the paraspinal muscles at L3 posteriorly.

Treatment: The PL3 tender point was treated on one occasion, in a position of comfort lasting approximately 7 minutes. As a result, the patient was able to increase his knee extension from -8° to -4° and his knee flexion from 25° to 125°, and he was able to bear much more weight on his right knee with less discomfort. The knee immobilizer was not used after the first visit. The patient returned for one more visit that week and two visits the next week, then was discharged after a total of four visits. One visit was used for positional release therapy and three visits for exercise prescription, at which time an exercise program to work on the mobility, flexibility, and strength of his knee, pelvis, and low back was started. This patient was off his crutches after the first visit and regained functional range of motion by his second visit.

This case study clearly indicates that if we had proceeded directly to the area of the patient's pain, his right knee, we would have found some tenderness to treat. However, the severity of tenderness at the knee was minor compared with the tenderness that the patient had in his low back. By following the general rules and principles and by treating the most dominant tender point, the effectiveness and efficiency of treatment was improved. The patient did have a low back problem as a result of the fall, and this dysfunction was affecting the muscles of his right lower extremity. This can be explained from the facilitated segment model discussed in Chapter 2.

Case Study 2 _____

Patient: Female in her early thirties.
Diagnosis: Medial collateral ligament strain, second degree, left knee.
Mechanism of injury: One week prior, patient fell and twisted her knee while skiing.
Weight-bearing status: Weight bearing as tolerated with crutches and knee immobilizer.
Range of motion: Extension -10°, knee flexion 30°.
Pain evaluation: Patient is in constant pain that varies in intensity. Most of the time she feels a lot of soreness and stiffness, approximately 5/10. It can get as high as 10/10 with sudden movement and movement beyond her available range.
Palpation: Swelling, heat, and tenderness noted on the medial aspect of the knee. On specific PRT evaluation, the dominant point was found to be the gluteus minimus, which is 1 cm lateral to the anterior inferior iliac spine. This point lies at the origin of the rectus femoris muscle.
Treatment: The gluteus minimus tender point was treated for approximately 6 minutes. As a result, knee extension was increased from -10° to -4° and knee flexion from 30° to 128°. This patient was able to get functional range of motion within the next 3 days and was able to tolerate full weight bearing without crutches or the knee immobilizer. Her therapy lasted another 3 weeks because she had some ligamentous damage, which gradually healed.

▌SUMMARY

These case studies show how two different people can have similar problems with range of motion, swelling, and pain in the knee. The source of their problem was two different regions. In the first case, it was coming from the low back; in the second case, it was coming from the pelvic region. A patient with knee pain may have the dominant point in the knee. In many cases, however, the dysfunction is completely removed from the area of pain. These cases reinforce the importance of a thorough evaluation of the patient to detect the location of the dysfunction instead of using pain as a guide. Remember that positional release therapy is only one mode of treatment. To improve the efficiency of treatment, incorporation of other treatment modalities is required. Various modalities are necessary to assist in the treatment of inflammation, atrophied muscles, and pain management. Other manual therapies may be needed to evaluate and treat articular or fascial tension. Finally, an exercise program should be instituted to improve strength, mobility, flexibility, cardiovascular fitness, and functional movement. The integration of the different modalities is discussed in more detail in Chapters 3 and 7.

6

Treatment Procedures

This chapter is divided into two sections. Section I covers the positional release therapy (PRT) assessment and treatment program for the upper half of the body: the cranium, the cervical spine, the thoracic spine and rib cage, and the upper limb. Section II deals with the same topics for the lumbar spine, pelvis, hip, sacrum, and lower limb. A scanning evaluation (SE) for the entire body can be found in the Appendix. The SE may be used once the student has mastered PRT for the whole body. In this chapter, separate SEs are provided for sections I and II, to allow the beginning student to be able to concentrate on one section at a time or so a local treatment may be performed, for example, for an acute injury.

Each major region of the body is introduced by a discussion of some of the clinical and functional considerations for the area of the body in question. This includes a perspective on pertinent functional anatomy, typical clinical manifestations, and special treatment considerations. Within each section the reader will find that separate areas of the body are headed by a drawing of the pertinent anatomy of the area showing the common tender points associated with that area. These subsections include the anterior cervical spine, the posterior cervical spine, the anterior thoracic spine, the knee, the shoulder, and so on.

Each treatment is associated with one or more tender points and is displayed on a single page. The treatment name is given with the appropriate abbreviation and the area of anatomy considered as being treated by that position of comfort (POC). This page includes a smaller drawing indicating the location of the specific tender points under consideration. A photograph or photographs demonstrate the commonly used techniques, and the text describes the techniques in detail, with variations that may be used in special circumstances or as preference dictates.

Note that tender points not directly over the tissue of involvement, which may be considered *reflex* points because they may be somewhat distant from the area of dysfunction, are designated with an asterisk (*).

In the Appendix, the reader will find an anatomic cross-reference that can help determine which treatment may be most pertinent to a given area of the body. There is also a cross reference of PRT terminology with that given by Jones.[9]

No text can hope to replace educational workshops. We encourage you to pursue the further development of your skills and to experiment with the technique and modify it to the needs of the presenting condition and to the greatest advantage of your patient.

¶DIAGNOSIS AND TREATMENT PROTOCOLS

The diagnosis of soft tissue involvement is based on several objective and subjective criteria. A careful history, including a clarification of any trauma or repetitive strain activities, is essential. It is important to differentiate non-musculoskeletal factors, such as viscerosomatic reflexes, malignancy, infectious processes, and psychologic involvement. Postural and structural asymmetry are significant indicators of involuntary antalgic strategies to reduce irritability of involved tissues. In general, an individual will adopt a posture that minimizes tension or loading of hypertonic or inflamed tissue.[9,23] Range-of-motion (ROM) assessment will help confirm and localize the involvement of flexors, extensors, rotators, lateral flexors, or related ligaments and fascia.[10] Local tissue changes (tension, texture, temperature, tenderness) and reduced joint play are also noted because these may indicate underlying dysfunction.[13] The *tender point* is a discrete, localized, hyperirritable region associated with the dysfunction and is used as a monitor during treatment.[21]

It is recommended that the user follow the outlined treatment positions as closely as possible because they have been carefully assessed over many years and have been determined to be efficacious in a large percentage of cases.

Once attempted, the user may then wish to adapt the technique to the needs of the individual if it is found that the prescribed method is less than satisfactory. The scanning evaluation will help the practitioner prioritize the treatment program.[4] We suggest that the practitioner use the following protocol for the most efficient use of this text:

1. Scan the patient's body for tender points and record them appropriately on the scanning evaluation.
2. Determine the most dominant tender point (DTP) using the general rules and principles.
3. Look up the appropriate treatment for the DTP. The page reference is provided in the scanning evaluation.
4. Treat according to the description provided in the treatment section in Chapter 6.

Treatment consists of precise positioning of the body part or joint in order to maximally relax the involved tissues. The descriptions of the positions of comfort are presented in their gross form. The ideal position is achieved through the use of micromovements, or fine-tuning.[8] This typically reduces the subjective tenderness and objective firmness of the associated tender point. Careful attention to the subtle changes occuring in the area of the tender point is necessary in order to obtain the optimal release. Once this ideal position is achieved, it is held for a period of no less than 90 seconds. During the positioning, which may last for 5 minutes or more, further softening, relaxation, pulsation, vibration, or *unwinding* of the tissues is often noted.

The positioning is followed by a passive return of the body part or joint to an anatomically neutral position. Reevaluation may then be carried out to confirm the efficacy of the therapeutic intervention. This approach will suffice for the majority of cases and will provide valuable experience in the development of the skills necessary to refine this art.

PRT Upper Quadrant Evaluation

Patient's name _____ Practitioner _____

Dates 1_____ 2_____ 3_____ 4_____ 5_____

● - Extremely sensitive   ◓ - Very sensitive   ◒ - Moderately sensitive   ○ - No tenderness

\ - Right   / - Left   + - Most sensitive   ⚲- Treatment

I.   Cranium (pages 43-63)

1. OM	○○○○○	6. DG	○○○○○	11. NAS	○○○○○	16. AT	○○○○○
2. OCC	○○○○○	7. MPT	○○○○○	12. SO	○○○○○	17. PT	○○○○○
3. PSB	○○○○○	8. LPT	○○○○○	13. FR	○○○○○	18. TPA	○○○○○
4. LAM	○○○○○	9. MAS	○○○○○	14. SAG	○○○○○	19. TPP	○○○○○
5. SH	○○○○○	10. MAX	○○○○○	15. LSB	○○○○○	_____	○○○○○

II.   Anterior, Medial, Lateral Cervical Spine (pages 65-76)

20. AC1	○○○○○	23. AC4	○○○○○	26. AC7	○○○○○	29. LC1	○○○○○
21. AC2	○○○○○	24. AC5	○○○○○	27. AC8	○○○○○	30. LC__	○○○○○
22. AC3	○○○○○	25. AC6	○○○○○	28. AMC	○○○○○	30. LC__	○○○○○

III.   Posterior Cervical Spine (pages 77-83)

31. PC1-F	○○○○○	34. PC3	○○○○○	37. PC6	○○○○○	_____	○○○○○
32. PC1-E	○○○○○	35. PC4	○○○○○	38. PC7	○○○○○	_____	○○○○○
33. PC2	○○○○○	36. PC5	○○○○○	39. PC8	○○○○○	_____	○○○○○

IV.   Anterior Thoracic Spine (pages 85-89)

40. AT1	○○○○○	43. AT4	○○○○○	46. AT7	○○○○○	49. AT10	○○○○○
41. AT2	○○○○○	44. AT5	○○○○○	47. AT8	○○○○○	50. AT11	○○○○○
42. AT3	○○○○○	45. AT6	○○○○○	48. AT9	○○○○○	51. AT12	○○○○○

V.   Anterior Ribs, Medial Ribs (pages 90-94)

52. AR1	○○○○○	57. AR6	○○○○○	62. MR3	○○○○○	67. MR8	○○○○○
53. AR2	○○○○○	58. AR7	○○○○○	63. MR4	○○○○○	68. MR 9	○○○○○
54. AR3	○○○○○	59. AR8	○○○○○	64. MR5	○○○○○	69. MR10	○○○○○
55. AR4	○○○○○	60. AR9	○○○○○	65. MR6	○○○○○	_____	○○○○○
56. AR5	○○○○○	61. AR10	○○○○○	66. MR7	○○○○○	_____	○○○○○

VI.   Posterior Thoracic Spine (pages 95-99)

70. PT1	○○○○○	73. PT4	○○○○○	76. PT7	○○○○○	79. PT10	○○○○○
71. PT2	○○○○○	74. PT5	○○○○○	77. PT8	○○○○○	80. PT11	○○○○○
72. PT3	○○○○○	75. PT6	○○○○○	78. PT9	○○○○○	81. PT12	○○○○○

VII. Posterior Ribs (pages 100-103)

82. PR1	○○○○○	85. PR4	○○○○○	88. PR7	○○○○○	91. PR10	○○○○○
83. PR2	○○○○○	86. PR5	○○○○○	89. PR8	○○○○○	92. PR11	○○○○○
84. PR3	○○○○○	87. PR6	○○○○○	90. PR9	○○○○○	93. PR12	○○○○○

VIII. Shoulder (pages 105-125)

94. TRA	○○○○○	99. SUB	○○○○○	104. PMI	○○○○○	109. ISS	○○○○○
95. SCL	○○○○○	100. SER	○○○○○	105. LD	○○○○○	110. ISM	○○○○○
96. AAC	○○○○○	101. MHU	○○○○○	106. PAC	○○○○○	111. ISI	○○○○○
97. SSL	○○○○○	102. BSH	○○○○○	107. SSM	○○○○○	112. TMA	○○○○○
98. BLH	○○○○○	103. PMA	○○○○○	108. MSC	○○○○○	113. TMI	○○○○○

IX. Elbow (pages 126-132)

114. LEP	○○○○○	116. RHS	○○○○○	118. MCD	○○○○○	120. MOL	○○○○○
115. MEP	○○○○○	117. RHP	○○○○○	119. LCD	○○○○○	121. LOL	○○○○○

X. Wrist & Hand (pages 133-137)

122. CFT	○○○○○	124. PWR	○○○○○	126. CM1	○○○○○	128. DIN	○○○○○
123. CET	○○○○○	125. DWR	○○○○○	127. PIN	○○○○○	129. IP	○○○○○

CRANIUM

¶ CRANIAL DYSFUNCTION

It is not within the scope of this text to delineate an exhaustive treatise on the complex functional anatomy of the cranium. The reader should refer to the resources listed in the Appendix to obtain training in this important and clinically relevant region. It is recommended that an anatomy text and the drawings at the beginning of this section be reviewed in order to familiarize oneself with the basic anatomic relationships.

For many practitioners, cranial lesions may present challenges in terms of diagnosis and treatment. Mobility and motility (self-actuated movement) within the cranium has now been well established, although it is not fully accepted in all circles. Sutherland,[19] Upledger,[22] and others have used various methods of diagnosis and treatment to normalize the function of this important area of the body. Cranial function may have a significant bearing on the circulation of the cerebrospinal fluid (CSF) to the central nervous system and thus on the functioning of the entire nervous system.[22] Dysfunctions caused by injuries, including birth trauma and persisting lesions resulting from childhood injuries, are not uncommon. Modern methods of birthing may have a significant effect on the prevalence of lateral strain lesions of the sphenoid and compression lesions of the temporoparietal suture.

Cranial dysfunction may manifest as headache, earache, tinnitus, vertigo, recurring sinusitis, lachrymal dysfunction, dental symptoms, dysphasia, temporomandibular joint (TMJ) dysfunction, seizure activity, and certain neurologic and cognitive conditions.[22]

With any cranial treatment, it is recommended that certain precautions be taken. Symptoms and signs of space-occupying lesions and acute head trauma are clear contraindications. A history of seizures or previous cerebrovascular accident should be approached with caution; if in doubt, a colleague with more experience in cranial therapy should be consulted.

The PRT approach to cranial therapy is precise and effective and can have an important role along with other techniques in the armementarium for addressing the cranial region.

¶ TREATMENT

Commonly used methods of cranial manipulation involve direct force against the movement barrier. Positional release therapy uses primarily indirect movement. Tender points are usually located in the vicinity of the cranial suture, with certain exceptions. The amount of force is in the range of 1 to 2 kg (2 to 5 lb).

CRANIUM *Tender Points*

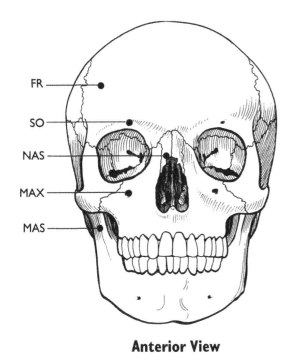

FR
SO
NAS
MAX
MAS

Anterior View

LAM
PSB
OCC
OM
SH
MPT
DG

Posterior View

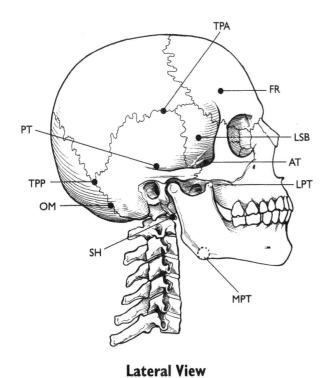

TPA
FR
PT
LSB
AT
LPT
TPP
OM
SH
MPT

Lateral View

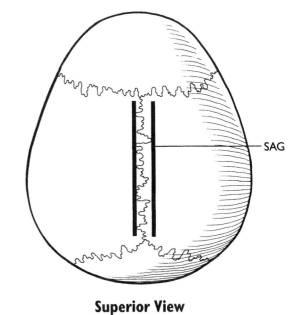

SAG

Superior View

CRANIUM

1. Occipitomastoid (OM)   Tentorium Cerebelli

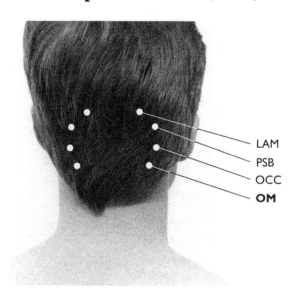

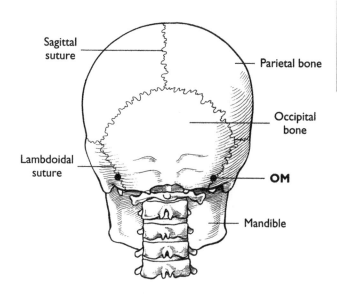

LAM
PSB
OCC
OM

Sagittal suture
Parietal bone
Occipital bone
Lambdoidal suture
OM
Mandible

| **Location of Tender Point** | This tender point is located on the occipitomastoid suture just medial and superior to the mastoid process. Pressure is applied anterosuperiorly. |

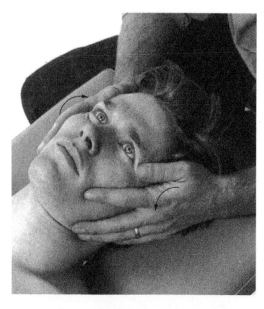

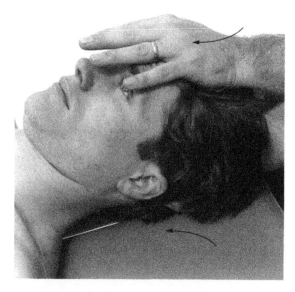

| **Position of Treatment** (Unilateral tenderness) | Patient lies supine. The therapist sits at the head of the table and grasps the cranium laterally with both palms. Pressure is applied medially, and counterrotation of both temporal bones is produced around a transverse axis. The direction of the rotary force is determined by the comfort of the patient or by the response of the tender point (which may be difficult to palpate). (See photo above left.) |

| **Position of Treatment** (Bilateral tenderness) | The patient lies supine. The therapist sits at the head of the table. The therapist grasps the occipital bone and applies an anterior and caudal pressure and with the other hand applies pressure posteriorly and caudally. The occipital hand exerts a greater force. (See photo above right.) |

2. Occipital (OCC)

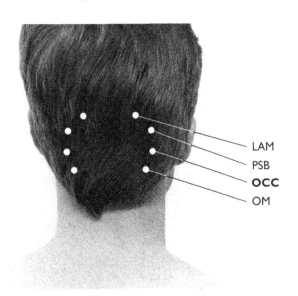

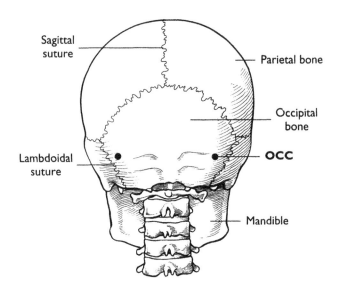

¶ **Location of Tender Point** This tender point is located medial to the lambdoid suture approximately 3 cm (1.2 in.) lateral to the posterior occipital protuberance just cephalad to the OM tender point. Pressure is applied anteriorly.

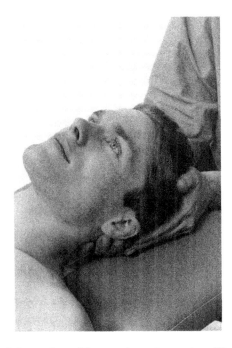

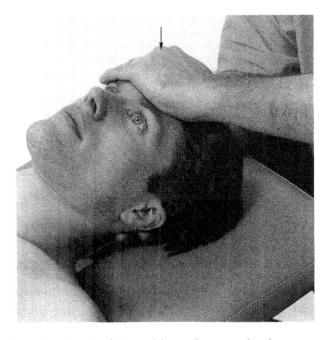

¶ **Position of Treatment** The patient is supine. The therapist is at the head of the table and grasps both mastoid processes with the heel and fingertips of the same hand or with the heels of both hands. Gentle pressure is applied medially. (See photo above left.)
Alternatively, the palpating hand is placed under the occiput, the other hand is placed on the anterior aspect of the frontal bone, and an anterior-posterior (AP) pressure is applied. (See photo above right.)

CRANIUM

3. Posterior Sphenobasilar (PSB)   Sphenobasilar Rotation

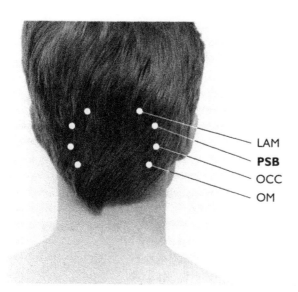

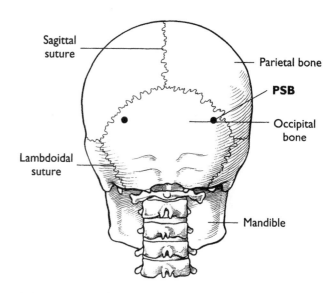

Location of Tender Point

This tender point is located just medial to the lambdoid suture approximately 3 cm (1.2 in.) superior to and 3 cm (1.2 in.) lateral and slightly superior to the posterior occipital protuberance. Pressure is applied anteriorly.

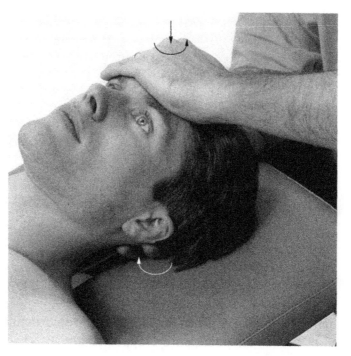

Position of Treatment

The patient is supine. The therapist sits at the head of the table and grasps the cranium with one hand on the frontal bone and one hand on the occipital bone. Pressure is exerted in a counterrotary direction around the AP axis. The direction of the rotation is determined by the comfort of the patient or by the response of the tender point (which may be difficult to palpate during the treatment).

4. Lambda (LAM)   Occipital Rotation

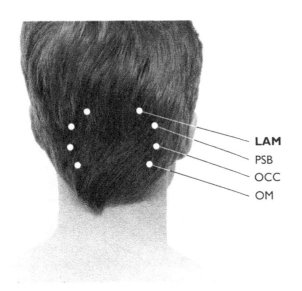

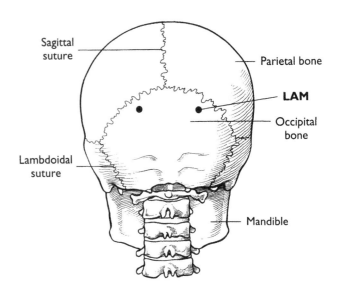

Sagittal suture

Parietal bone

LAM

Occipital bone

Lambdoidal suture

Mandible

LAM
PSB
OCC
OM

Location of Tender Point   This tender point is located medial to the lambdoid suture approximately 2 cm (0.8 in.) inferior to the lambda. Pressure is applied anteriorly.

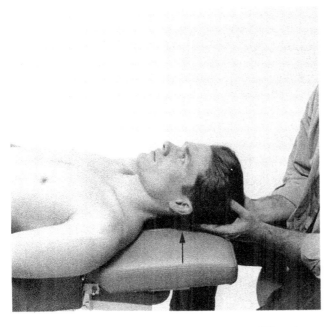

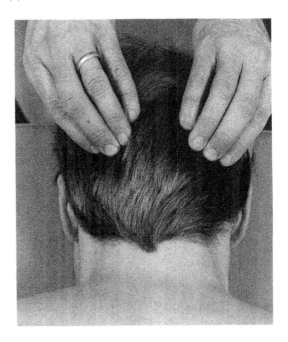

Position of Treatment   The patient is supine. The therapist applies anterior pressure to the occipital bone, at the level of the tender point, on the opposite side.

CRANIUM

5. Stylohyoid (SH)

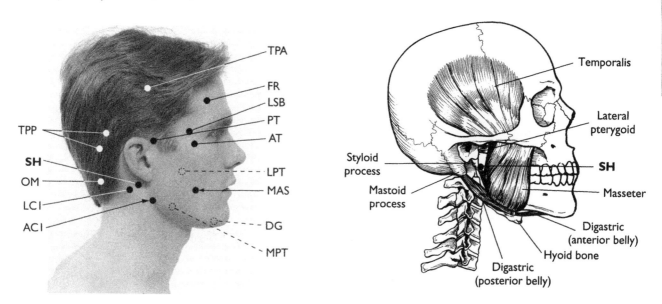

Location of Tender Point   This tender point is located on the styloid process just anterior and medial to the mastoid process (pressure is medial).

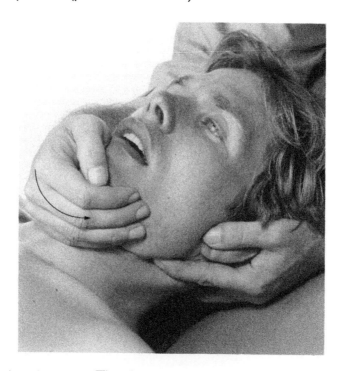

Position of Treatment   The patient is supine. The therapist flexes the upper cervical spine, opens the patient's mouth, and pushes the mandible toward the tender point side.
Alternatively, the hyoid bone is pushed from the opposite side toward the tender point side (not shown).

6. Digastric (DG)

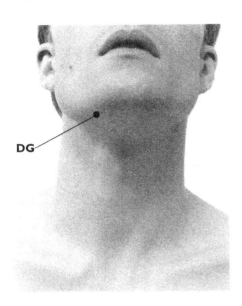

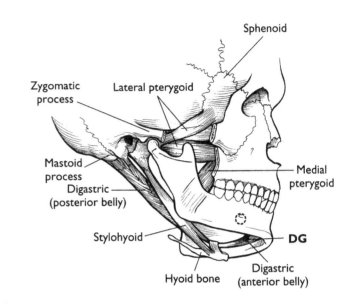

■ **Location of**
  Tender Point   This tender point is located in the anterior belly of the digastric muscle just medial to the inferior ramus of the mandible and anterior to the angle of the mandible. Pressure is applied in a cephalad direction.

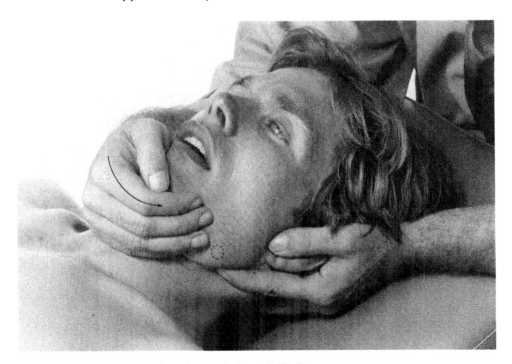

■ **Position of**
  Treatment   The treatment is that for stylohyoid (SH).
  Alternatively, the hyoid bone is pushed from the opposite side toward the tender point side (not shown).

CRANIUM

7. Medial Pterygoid (MPT)

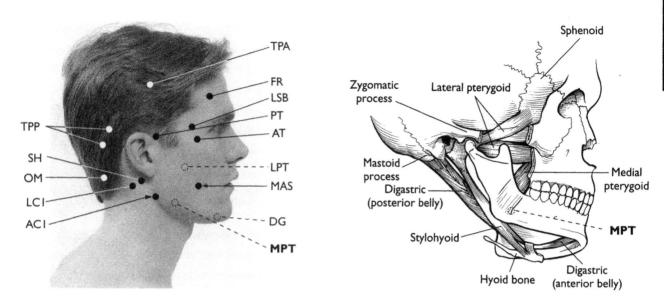

Location of Tender Point   This tender point is located on the medial surface of the ascending ramus of the mandible, just superior to the mandibular angle. Pressure is applied laterally.

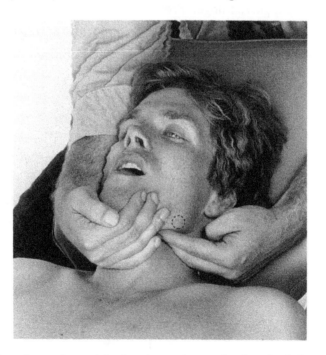

Position of Treatment   The patient is supine with the therapist at the head of the table. The therapist pushes the mandible away from the tender point side while applying a stabilizing force on the contralateral side of the frontal bone.

Note: This point is found inferior and medial to ACI.

8. Lateral Pterygoid (LPT)

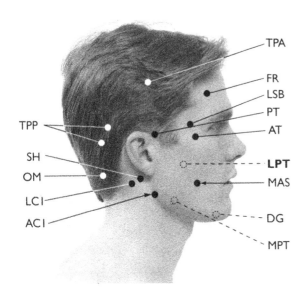

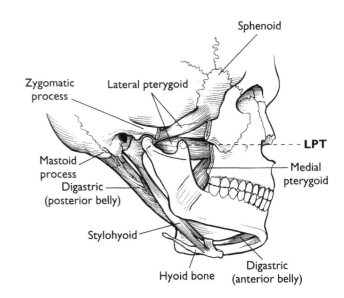

■ **Location of Tender Point**

1. Intraorally, medial to the coronoid process of the mandible in the posterior and superior aspect of the cheek pouch on the lateral aspect of the lateral pterygoid plate. Use a gloved finger. Pressure is applied posteriorly.

2. Extraorally, with the mouth slightly open, just anterior to the articular process of the mandible and inferior to the zygomatic arch.

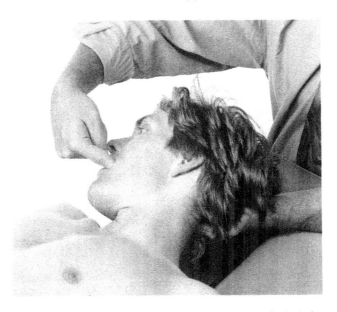

■ **Position of Treatment**

The patient lies supine. The patient's jaw is opened slightly and the head is supported and placed in a position moderate flexion, rotation, and side bending away from the tender point side.

Note: This position is similar to the treatment for AC3.

CRANIUM

9. Masseter (MAS)   Masseter, Temporalis

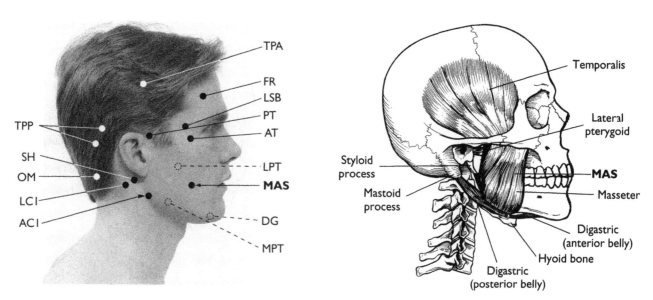

Location of Tender Point   This tender point is located on the anterior border of the masseter muscle over the anterior edge of ascending ramus of the mandible. Pressure is applied posteriorly.

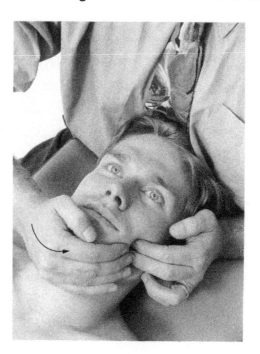

Position of Treatment   The patient is supine. The therapist braces the patient's head against the therapist's chest. The jaw is pushed toward the side of the tender point, and closure pressure is applied on the mandible toward the tender point side while applying a counterforce on the ipsilateral aspect of the frontal bone toward the opposite side.

10. Maxilla (MAX)

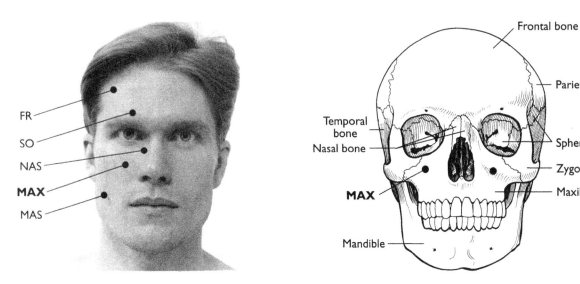

FR
SO
NAS
MAX
MAS

Frontal bone
Parietal bone
Temporal bone
Nasal bone
Sphenoid bone
Zygomatic bone
Maxilla
MAX
Mandible

| **Location of Tender Point** | This tender point is located in the region of the infraorbital foramen. Pressure is applied posteriorly. |

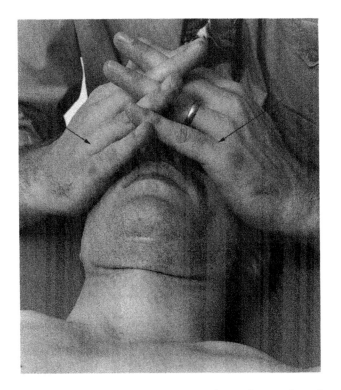

| **Position of Treatment** | The patient is supine. The therapist interlaces his or her fingers and compresses medially with the heels of both hands on the zygomatic portion of the maxillary bones. |

CRANIUM

11. Nasal (NAS)   Internasal Suture

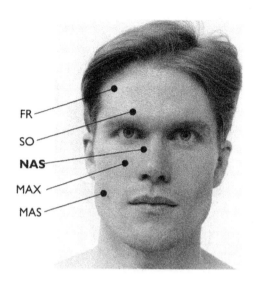

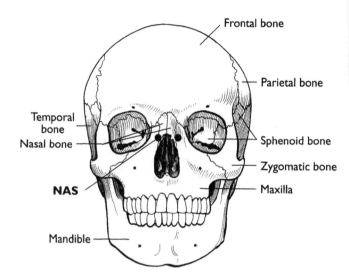

Location of Tender Point   This tender point is located on the anterolateral aspect of the nose. Pressure is applied posteromedially.

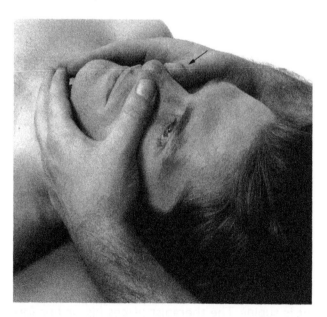

Position of Treatment   The patient is supine. The therapist pushes medially on the portion of the nose contralateral to the tender point.

12. Supraorbital (SO)   Frontonasal Joint

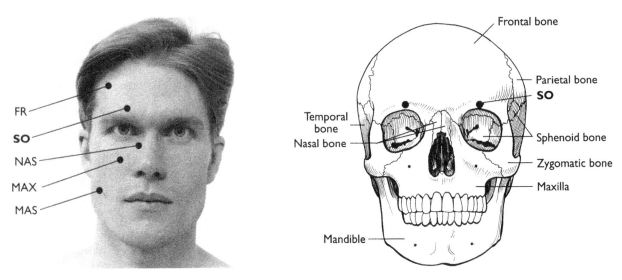

Frontal bone
Parietal bone
SO
Temporal bone
Nasal bone
Sphenoid bone
Zygomatic bone
Maxilla
Mandible

FR
SO
NAS
MAX
MAS

| **Location of Tender Point** | This tender point is located in the region of the supraorbital foramen. Pressure is applied posteriorly. |

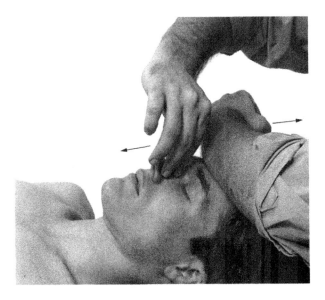

| **Position of Treatment** | The patient is supine. The therapist places his or her forearm on the patient's forehead and pulls in a cephalad direction while pinching the nasal bones with the fingers of the other hand and pulling in a caudad direction. |

CRANIUM

13. Frontal (FR)

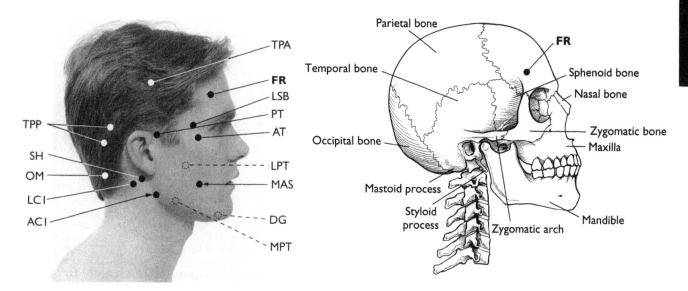

Location of Tender Point This tender point is located above the lateral portion of the orbit on the frontal bone. Pressure is applied medially.

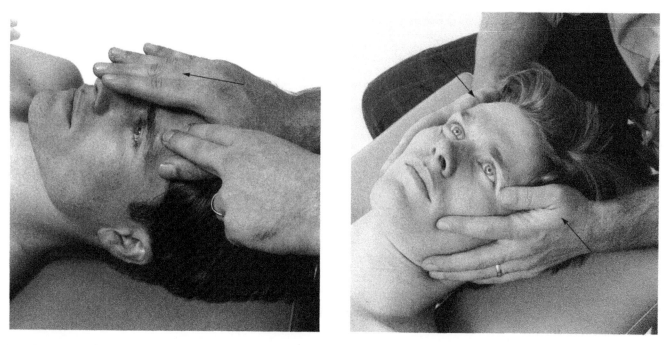

Position of Treatment The patient is supine. The therapist pushes the top of the frontal bone caudally (see photo above left) or compresses the frontal bone bilaterally (see photo above right).

14. Sagittal Suture (SAG)   Falx Cerebri

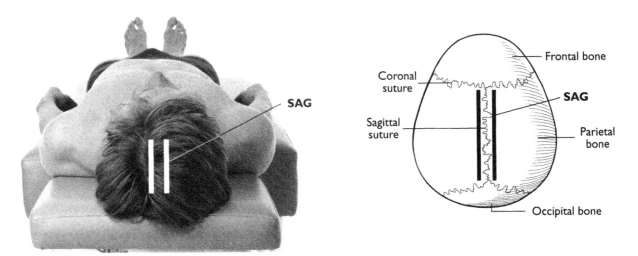

Location of Tender Point	This tender point is located on the superior aspect of the head just lateral to and along either side of the sagittal suture. Pressure is applied caudally.

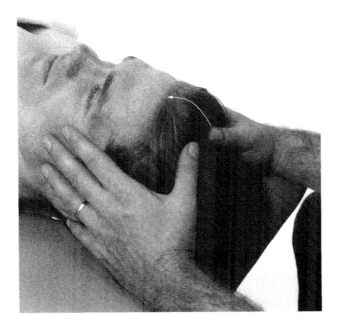

Position of Treatment	The patient is supine. The therapist pushes caudally on the parietal bone just lateral to the sagittal suture on the opposite side of the tender point.

CRANIUM

15. Lateral Sphenobasilar (LSB)   Sphenobasilar Lateral Strain

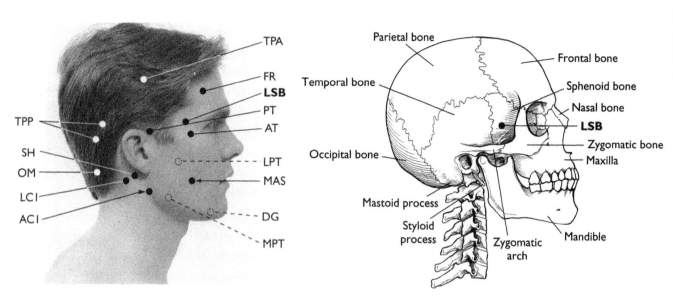

Location of Tender Point   This tender point is located on the lateral aspect of the greater wing of the sphenoid in a depression behind the lateral ridge of the orbit. Pressure is applied medially.

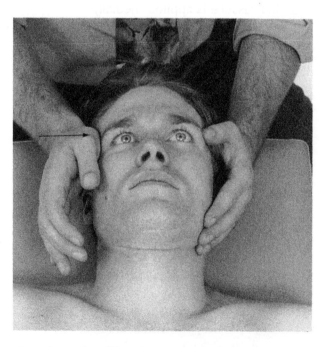

Position of Treatment   The patient is supine. The therapist applies a lateral pressure on the opposite greater wing of the sphenoid toward the tender point side. A counterpressure is used on the frontal bone and the zygoma of the involved side using the fingers and heel of the hand.

16. Anterior Temporalis (AT)

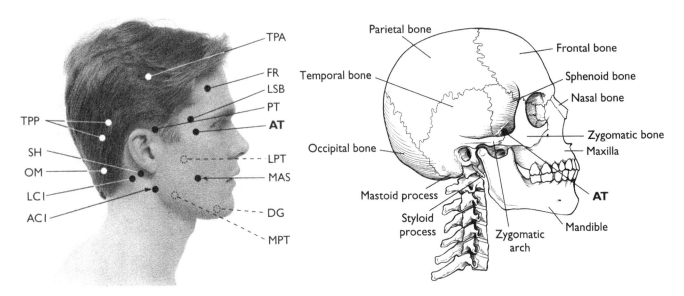

■ **Location of Tender Point**   This tender point is located in the anterior fibers of the temporalis muscle approximately 2 cm (0.8 in.) posterior and lateral to the orbit of the eye and superior to the zygomatic arch. Pressure is applied medially.

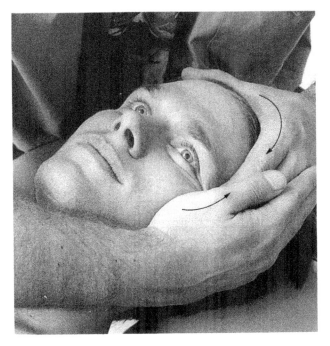

■ **Position of Treatment**   The patient is supine. The therapist is on the side of the tender point and grasps the frontal bone with one hand and applies a force around an AP axis toward the tender point. The heel of the other hand is placed under the zygomatic bone, and pressure is exerted in a cephalad direction.

CRANIUM

17. Posterior Temporalis (PT)

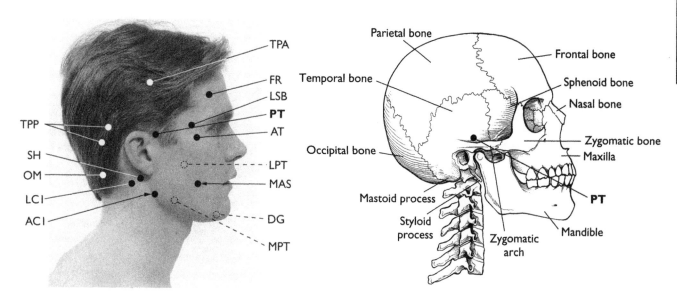

Location of Tender Point This tender point is located in the posterior fibers of the temporalis muscle approximately 3 cm (1.2 in.) anterior to the external auditory meatus superior to the zygomatic arch. Pressure is applied medially.

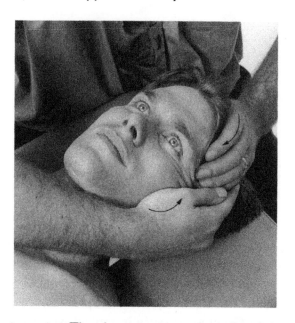

Position of Treatment The patient is supine. The therapist is on the side of the tender point, grasps the parietal bone with one hand, and applies a force to rotate the skull around an AP axis toward the tender point. The heel of the other hand is placed under the zygomatic bone, and pressure is applied in a cephalad direction.

Note: AT and PT are treated using a similar technique.

18. Temporoparietal (Anterior) (TPA)

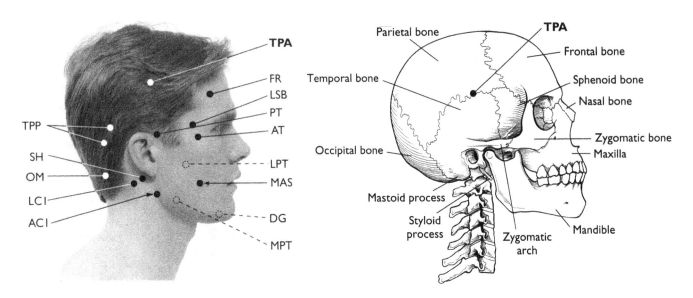

| | Location of Tender Point | This tender point is located cephalad to the ear, on or just above the temporoparietal suture. Pressure is applied medially. |

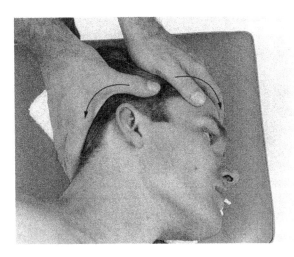

Position of Treatment (Unilateral tenderness)   The patient lies on the unaffected side with a small roll under the opposite zygomatic area. The therapist sits near the head of the patient, grasps the parietal bone with the fingers, and pulls the parietal bone cephalad and medially away from the tender point side. Alternatively, the therapist may stand and apply the force with the heel of the hand. Counterpressure is applied with the other hand in a medial direction on the mastoid process on the same side as the tender point.

Position of Treatment (Bilateral tenderness)   The patient is supine with the therapist seated at the head of the table. The therapist grasps the patient's cranium on both sides, just cephalad to the temporoparietal suture on the parietal bones. A medial pressure is applied bilaterally (see bottom right photo on p. 57).

CRANIUM

19. Temporoparietal (Posterior) (TPP)

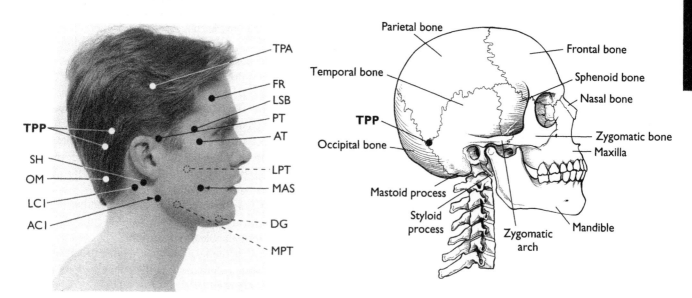

Location of Tender Point   This tender point is located at the junction of the lambdoid the temporoparietal sutures approximately 3 cm (1.2 in.) posterior to the external auditory meatus, in a depression on the skull. Pressure is applied medially.

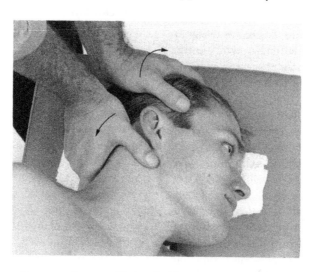

Position of Treatment
(Unilateral tenderness)   The patient lies on the unaffected side with a small roll under the opposite zygomatic area. The therapist applies a force superior to the tender point, on the parietal bone, in a cephalad and medial direction in order to rotate the skull away from the tender point side. Counterpressure is applied medially on the ipsilateral mastoid process with the other hand.

Position of Treatment
(Bilateral tenderness)   The patient lies supine with the therapist at the head of the table. The therapist applies bilateral compression with the palms on both sides of the skull posterior to the ears (see bottom right photo on p. 57).

CERVICAL SPINE

CERVICAL DYSFUNCTION

Bipedal posture has afforded human beings numerous evolutionary advantages, including an increased range of visual surveillance of the surroundings and an improved ability to manipulate the materials in the environment. However, the raised center of gravity also causes greater translational forces and resultant trauma to the postural supportive tissues. The head and neck are particularly vulnerable to horizontal forces, which can be induced by falls or blows to the body. The relatively large mass of the head is a source of significant inertial force in the event of trauma to the cervical region. The bane of modern existence, the automobile, provides unique opportunities for especially severe trauma to the relatively delicate supportive elements of the cervical spine. Paraspinal muscles in the anterior, posterior, and lateral compartments; the suboccipital musculature; the paravertebral, capsular, and ligamentous elements; and the superficial fascia may be variously compromised depending on the direction and magnitude of the displacing forces.[17]

It appears that the deep, intrinsic tissues related to the intervertebral segment are the particular focus of persisting dysfunction, and it is to this level that therapeutic interest is directed.[1] The multifidus and rotatores posteriorly, the scalenes anteriorly and laterally, the longus capitis and longus colli anteriorly, and the suboccipitals are the active tissues that have the greatest segmental motor and sensory effect on the cervical spine.[11] Palpation of the tender points on the posterior, inferior aspect of the spinous processes may necessitate slight flexion of the neck, and both sides of the bifid process should be examined.

Clinical expressions of cervical dysfunction include neck pain, restriction of cervical motion, upper limb symptoms (pain, paresthesia, paresis), upper thoracic pain, headaches, dysphagia, nonproductive cough, vertigo, and tinnitus. The neck seems especially prone to stress-related responses and patients who are anxious should be evaluated for psychologic factors.[16] Headache patterns, according to Jones,[9] follow a segmental pattern, with C1,2 associated with frontal headache, C3,4 with lateral head pain, C4 with occipital pain, and C5 with whole head pain. Jones[9] also points out that dysfunction at the level of C3 is often associated with earache, tinnitus, or vertigo.[9] Upper limb involvement may be traced to dermatomal patterns associated with the nerve root distribution of the brachial plexus.

To locate specific segments of the cervical spine, the following list of landmarks may be a helpful guide:

C1: Transverse process just inferior to mastoid process and posterior to the earlobe.

C2: Spinous process is located approximately 1.5 to 2 cm (0.6 to 0.8 in.) inferior to the midline of the occiput. This is a wide, bifid spinous process.

C3: Located at the level of the hyoid anteriorly. On extension, spinous process remains palpable.

C4: Located at the level of the superior border of the thyroid cartilage anteriorly. On extension, spinous process is not palpable.

C5: Located at the level of the inferior border of the thyroid cartilage anteriorly. Spinous process remains palpable on extension.

C6: Located at the level of the cricoid cartilage anteriorly. Spinous process is easily palpable on extension and is often bifid.

C7: Prominent bifid spinous process. To differentiate from T1, perform cervical extension. The C7 spinous moves anteriorly more than T1.[3,14]

TREATMENT

Positioning of the cervical spine involves using the tender point as a fulcrum about which all of the component movements (flexion, extension, rotation, and lateral flexion) are focused. Treatment of anterior lesions consists of precise flexion of the cervical spine at the level of the tender point. With scalene involvement, the addition of contralateral rotation and a variable amount of lateral flexion are also induced. Posterior dysfunction may involve the posterior suboccipitals, multifidus, or rotatores. These are treated using varying degrees of extension and often the addition of rotation and lateral flexion away from the tender point side. Occipital flexion, by retracting the patient's mandible, should be maintained throughout any positions involving cervical extension. The sternocleidomastoid may need to be pushed laterally or medially in order to palpate the anterior tender points. The patient's neck should be relaxed during palpation and treatment.

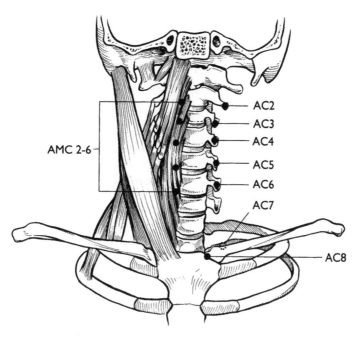

AC2
AC3
AC4
AC5
AC6
AC7
AC8

AMC 2-6

Anterior View

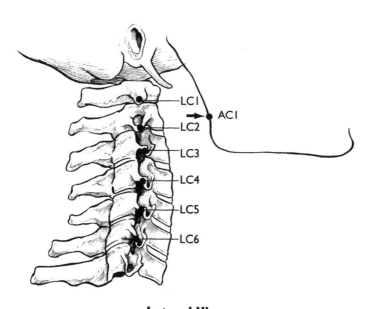

LCI
LC2
LC3
LC4
LC5
LC6

ACI

Lateral View

20. Anterior First Cervical (AC1)   Rectus Capitis Anterior

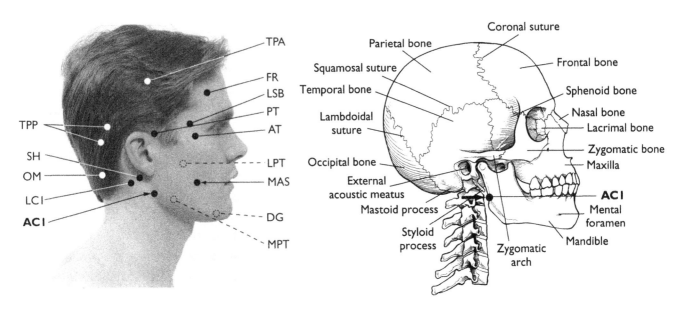

Location of Tender Point
This tender point is located on the posterior aspect of the ascending ramus of the mandible approximately 1 cm (0.4 in.) superior to the angle of the mandible. Pressure is applied anteriorly.

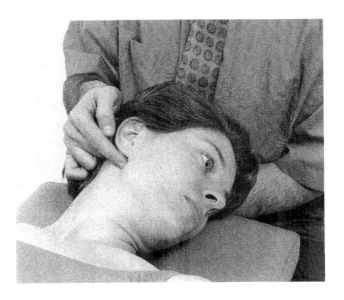

Position of Treatment
The patient lies supine with the therapist sitting at the head of the table. The therapist grasps the sides of the patient's head and rotates the head markedly away from the tender point side. Fine-tuning may include slight cervical flexion, extension, or lateral flexion.

21. Anterior Second Cervical (AC2)   Longus Colli

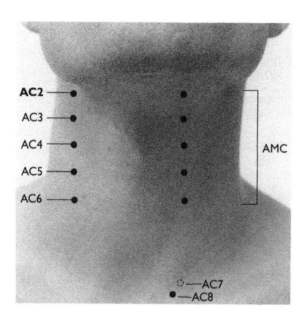

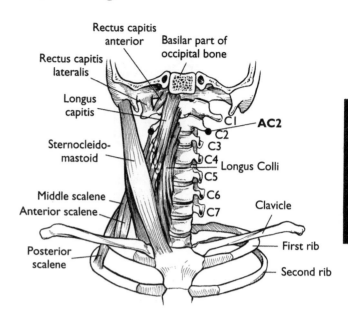

Location of Tender Point   This tender point is located on the anterior surface of the tip of the transverse process of C2. This is located approximately 1 cm (04 in.) inferior to the tip of the mastoid process. Pressure is applied posteromedially.

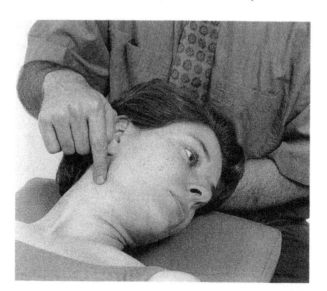

Position of Treatment   The patient is supine with the therapist sitting at the head of the table. The therapist grasps the sides of the patient's head and rotates the head markedly away from the tender point side. This treatment is similar to that for AC1 except that slightly more flexion is used.

22. Anterior Third Cervical (AC3)   Longus Capitis, Longus Colli

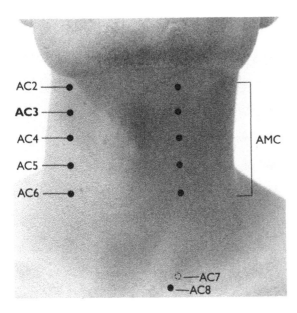

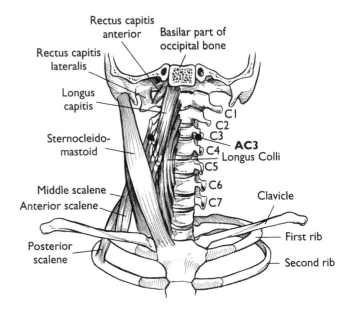

Location of Tender Point   This tender point is located on the anterior surface of the tip of the transverse process of C3 at the level of the hyoid. This area may usually be found directly posterior to the angle of the mandible. Pressure is applied posteromedially.

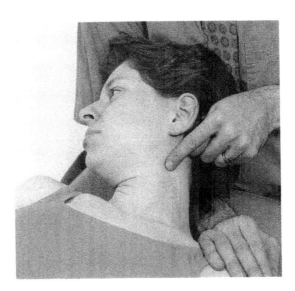

Position of Treatment   The patient lies supine with the therapist sitting at the head of the table. The therapist grasps the patient's head and produces marked flexion to the level of C3, rotation away from the tender point side, and lateral flexion away from or toward the tender point side.

Note: The therapist may support the head on the therapist's forearm by passing it under the head from the non-tender point side and resting the palm of the hand on the patient's anterior shoulder on the tender point side.

23. Anterior Fourth Cervical (AC4)   Scalenus Ant., Longus Capitis, Longus Colli

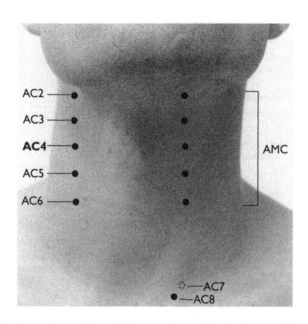

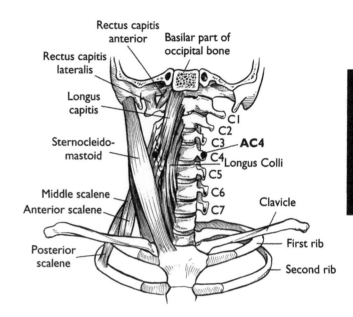

Location of Tender Point   This tender point is located on the anterior surface of the tip of the transverse process of C4 at the level of the superior border of the thyroid cartilage. This area is usually found just inferior and posterior to the angle of the mandible. Pressure is applied posteromedially.

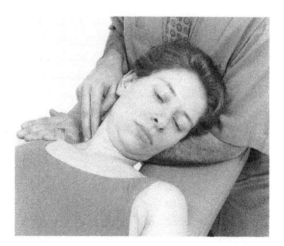

Position of Treatment   The patient lies supine with the therapist sitting at the head of the table. The therapist grasps the patient's head and produces moderate cervical flexion to the level of C4 (cervical extension may be required for this segment), rotation, and lateral flexion away from the tender point side.

Note: The therapist may support the head on the therapist's forearm by passing it under the head from the non-tender point side and resting the palm of the hand on the patient's anterior shoulder on the tender point side.

24. Anterior Fifth Cervical (AC5)   Scalenus Ant., Longus Capitis, Longus Colli

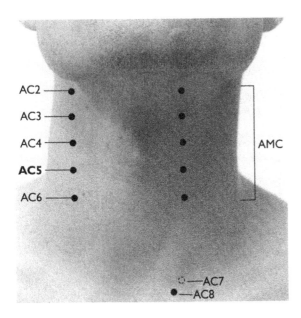

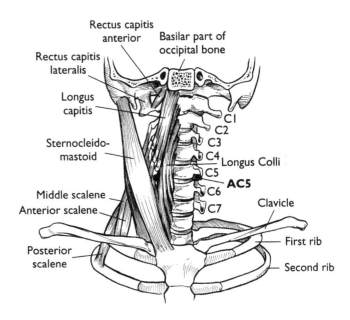

| Location of Tender Point | This tender point is located on the anterior surface of the tip of the transverse process of C5 at the level of the inferior border of the thyroid cartilage. Pressure is applied posteromedially. |

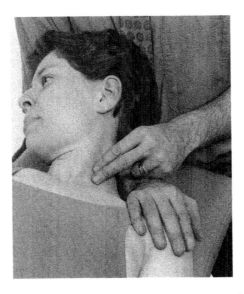

| Position of Treatment | The patient lies supine with the therapist sitting at the head of the table. The therapist grasps the patient's head and produces cervical flexion down to the level of the tender point and rotation and lateral flexion away from the tender point side. |

Note: The therapist may support the head on the therapist's forearm by passing it under the head from the non-tender point side and resting the palm of the hand on the patient's anterior shoulder on the tender point side.

25. Anterior Sixth Cervical (AC6)   Scalenus Ant., Longus Colli

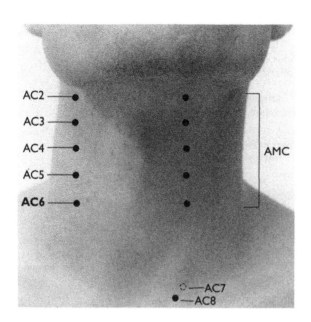

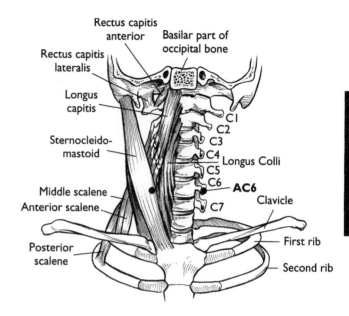

| **Location of Tender Point** | This tender point is located on the anterior surface of the tip of the transverse process of C6 at the level of the cricoid cartilage. Pressure is applied posteromedially. |

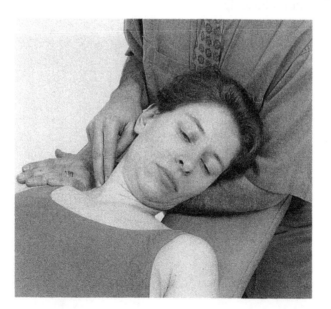

| **Position of Treatment** | The patient lies supine with the therapist sitting at the head of the table. The therapist grasps the patient's head and produces cervical flexion down to the level of the tender point and rotation and lateral flexion away from the tender point side. |

Note: The therapist may support the head on the therapist's forearm by passing it under the head from the non-tender point side and resting the palm of the hand on the patient's anterior shoulder on the tender point side.

CERVICAL SPINE

26. Anterior Seventh Cervical (AC7)   Sternocleidomastoid

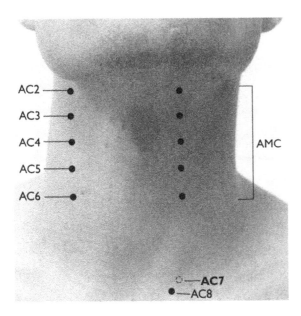

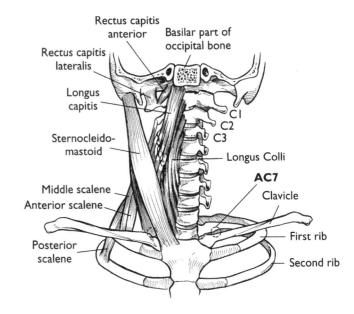

| **Location of Tender Point** | This tender point is located on the posterior superior surface of the clavicle approximately 3 cm (1.2 in.) lateral to the medial head of the clavicle. Pressure is applied anteriorly and inferiorly. |

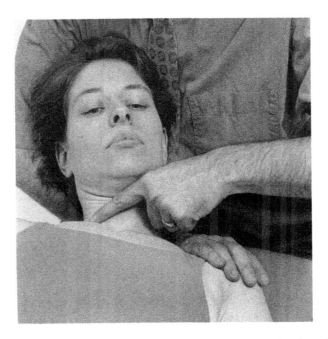

| **Position of Treatment** | The patient lies supine with the therapist sitting at the head of the table. The therapist supports the patient's midcervical area and markedly flexes and laterally flexes the cervical spine toward the tender point side, rotating the cervical spine slightly away from the tender point side. |

27. Anterior Eighth Cervical (AC8)   Sternohyoid, Omohyoid

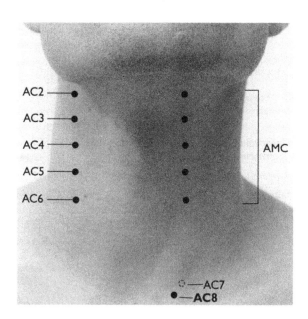

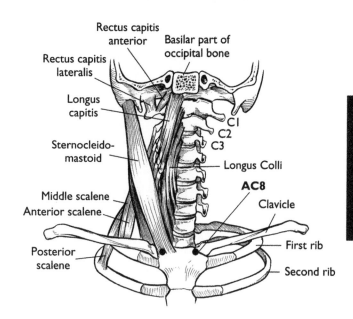

Location of Tender Point   This tender point is located on the medial surface of the proximal head of the clavicle. Pressure is applied laterally.

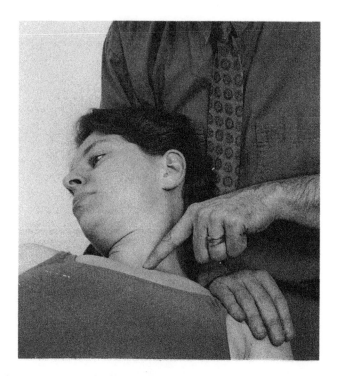

Position of Treatment   The patient lies supine with the therapist at the head of the table. The therapist grasps the patient's head and flexes the cervical spine slightly, laterally flexes slightly away from the tender point side, and rotates markedly away from the tender point side.

CERVICAL SPINE

28. Anterior Medial Cervical (AMC)   Longus Colli, Infrahyoid

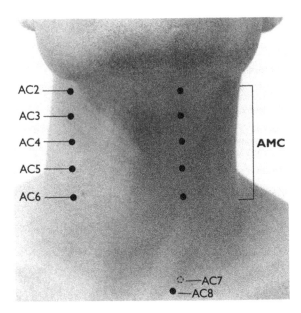

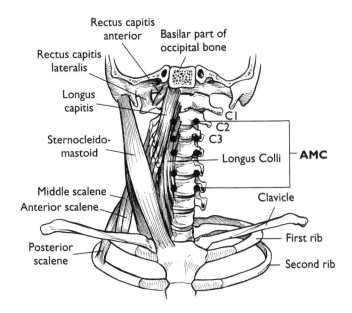

▌ **Location of Tender Point**   These tender points are found along the lateral aspect of the trachea. The trachea is pushed slightly to the side to palpate the point. Pressure is applied posteriorly.

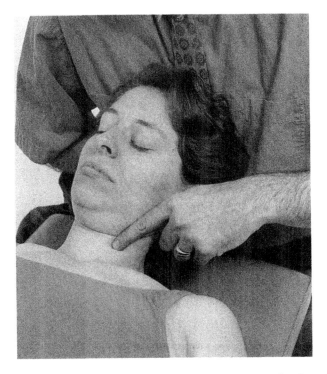

▌ **Position of Treatment**   The patient lies supine with the therapist sitting at the head of the table. The therapist grasps the patient's head and markedly flexes the neck while adding slight side bending toward and rotation away from the tender point side.

LATERAL CERVICAL

29. Lateral First Cervical (LC1)   Rectus Capitis Lateralis

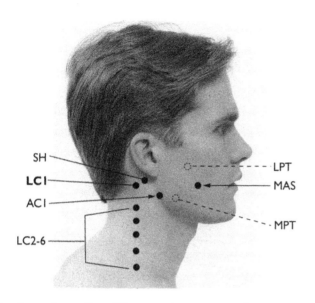 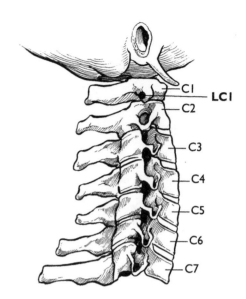

Location of Tender Point   This tender point is located on the lateral aspect of the transverse process of C1. Pressure is applied medially.

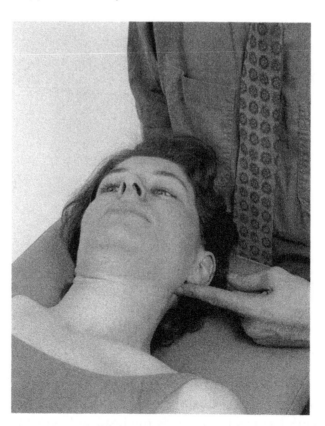

Position of Treatment   The patient is supine with the therapist sitting at the table. The therapist grasps the patient's head and laterally flexes the head toward or away from the tender point side depending on the response of the tissues.

30. Lateral Cervical (LC2-6) Scalenus Medius

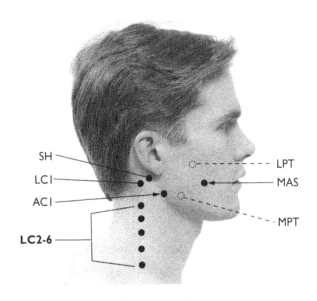

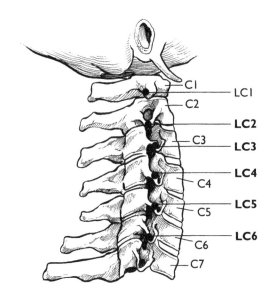

| **Location of Tender Point** | These tender points are located on the lateral aspect of the articular processes of the cervical vertebrae. Pressure is applied medially. |

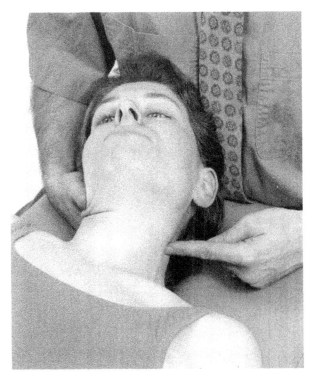

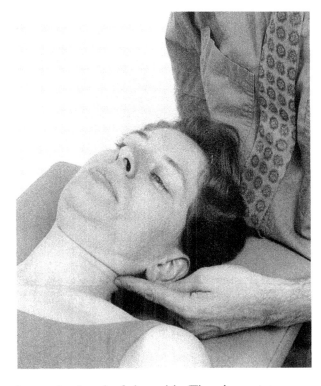

| **Position of Treatment** | The patient is supine with the therapist at the head of the table. The therapist grasps the patient's head and side bends the head and neck toward or away from the tender point side depending on the response of the tissues. Flexion, extension, or rotation may be needed to fine-tune the position. |

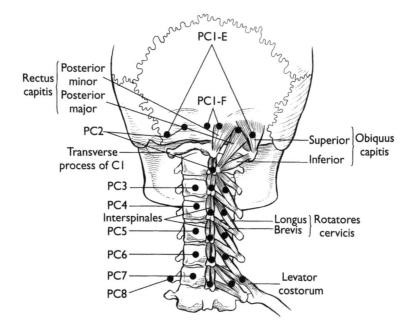

PC1-E

Rectus capitis { Posterior minor / Posterior major

PC1-F

PC2

Transverse process of C1

Superior / Inferior } Obiquus capitis

PC3

PC4

Interspinales

Longus / Brevis } Rotatores cervicis

PC5

PC6

PC7

PC8

Levator costorum

31. Posterior First Cervical—Flexion (PC1-F)
Rectus Capitis Anterior

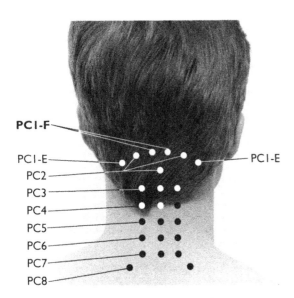

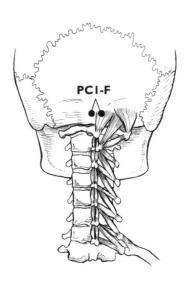

Location of Tender Point This tender point is located on the base of the skull on the medial side of the insertion of the semispinalis capitis approximately 3 cm (1.2 in.) inferior to the posterior occipital protuberance. Pressure is applied laterally and superiorly.

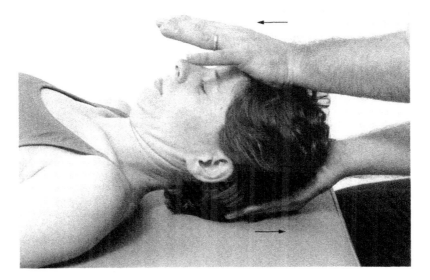

Position of Treatment The patient lies supine with the therapist sitting at the head of the table. The therapist grasps the patient's head by putting one hand on the occiput and pulling in a cephalad direction and the other hand on the frontal bone pushing caudad. This will create marked occipital flexion. Fine-tuning may include slight side bending toward and rotation away from the tender point side.

CERVICAL SPINE

32. Posterior First Cervical—Extension (PC1-E)
Obliquus Capitis Superior

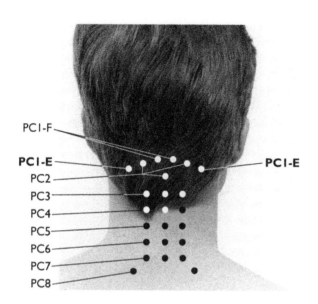

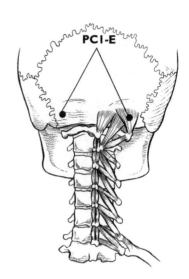

Location of Tender Point   This tender point is located on a flat portion of the occipital bone approximately 1 to 1.5 cm (0.4 to 0.6 in.) medial to the mastoid process. Pressure is applied in a cephalad direction.

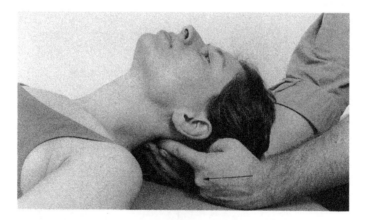

Position of Treatment   The patient lies supine with the head resting on the table. The therapist sits at the head of the table. The therapist then places the hand under the patient's head with the fingers pointing caudally. With pressure from the heel of the hand, the therapist pushes caudally on the head in such a manner as to induce a local extension of the occiput on C1. The therapist can also add moderate rotation and slight side bending away from the tender point side to fine-tune.

Note: One hand may be used to palpate the tender point and to apply caudal pressure on the top of the posterior aspect of the head; the other hand is positioned on the frontal bone to assist the movement (not shown).

33. Posterior Second Cervical (PC2) Rectus Capitis Posterior Major/Minor

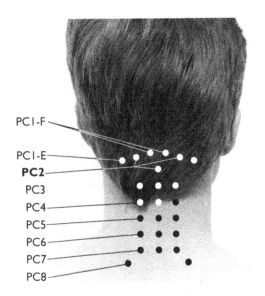

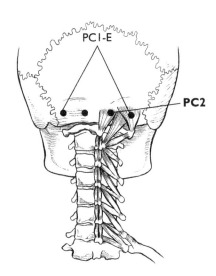

▪ Location of Tender Point This tender point is located on the base of the skull on the lateral side of the insertion of the semispinalis capitis. Pressure is applied medially and superiorly. Another tender point may be found on the superior surface of the spinous process of C2. Pressure is applied inferiorly.

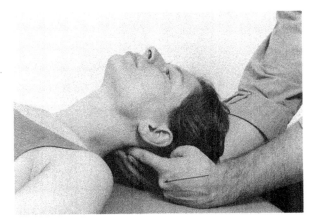

▪ Position of Treatment The patient lies supine with the head resting on the table. The therapist sits at the head of the table. The therapist then places the hand under the patient's head with the fingers pointing caudally. With pressure from the heel of the hand, the therapist pushes caudally on the head in such a manner as to induce a local extension of the occiput on C1. The therapist can also add moderate rotation and slight side bending away from the tender point side to fine-tune.

Note: One hand may be used to palpate the tender point and to apply caudal pressure on the top of the posterior aspect of the head; the other hand is positioned on the frontal bone to assist the movement (not shown).

34. Posterior Third Cervical (PC3)
Rotatores, Multifidus, Interspinalis

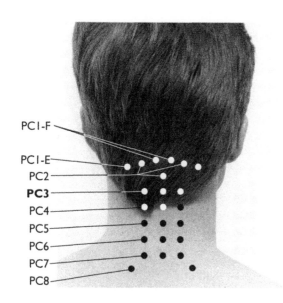

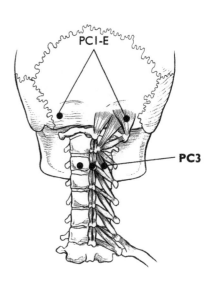

| Location of Tender Point | This tender point is located on the inferior surface of the spinous process of C2 (pressure applied superiorly) or on the articular process of C3 (pressure applied anteriorly). Slight flexion may be needed to allow the tender point to be accessible. |

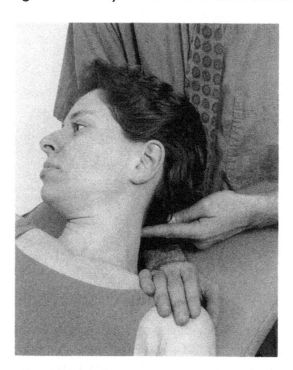

| Position of Treatment | The patient lies supine with the therapist sitting at the head of the table. The therapist grasps the patient's head and extends the cervical spine to the level of C3 and laterally flexes and rotates it away from the tender point side. This lesion may require flexion, in which case the treatment is identical to that for AC3. |

35-38. Posterior Fourth, Fifth, Sixth, and Seventh Cervical
(PC4-7)   Rotatores, Multifidus, Interspinalis

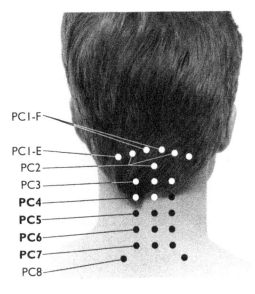
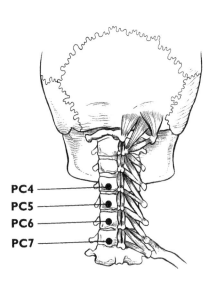

Location of	This tender point is located on the inferior surface of the spinous process of verte-

**Location of
Tender Point**   This tender point is located on the inferior surface of the spinous process of verte-brae above (pressure applied superiorly) or on the articular process of the involved vertebral segment (pressure applied anteriorly). Slight flexion may be needed to allow the tender point to be accessible.

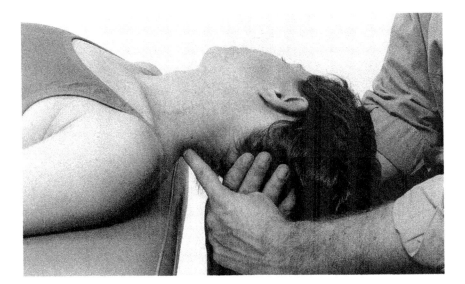

**Position of
Treatment**   The patient lies supine with the therapist sitting at the head of the table. The thera-pist grasps the patient's head and extends it moderately and laterally flexes and rotates it away from the tender point side. Extension is increased progressively as one treats progressively caudal lesions.

39. Posterior Eighth Cervical (PC8)   Levator Costorum

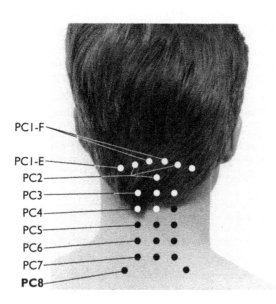

PC1-F
PC1-E
PC2
PC3
PC4
PC5
PC6
PC7
PC8

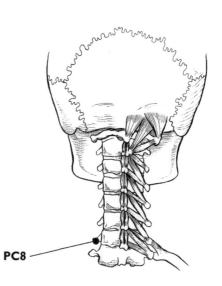

PC8

Location of Tender Point

The therapist palpates anterior to the upper portion of the trapezius to locate the upper border of the first rib. The tender point is found by palpating medially toward the base of the neck until the transverse process of C7 is encountered and then moving onto the posterosuperior surface of the transverse process. Pressure is applied anteriorly on the posterior surface of the transverse process of C7.

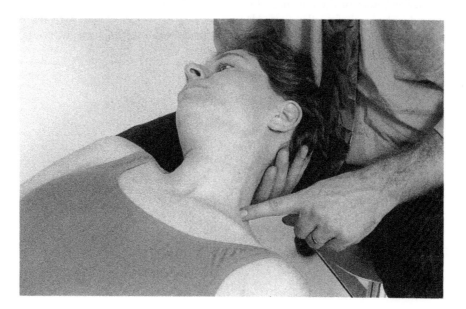

Position of Treatment

The patient lies supine with the therapist sitting at the head of the table. The therapist grasps the patient's head and induces marked lateral flexion and slight rotation away from the tender point side along with slight cervical extension.

CERVICAL SPINE

THORACIC SPINE AND RIB CAGE _____

¶THORACIC DYSFUNCTION

The thoracic spine and rib cage contain no less than 84 synovial joints. They form a protective housing for several vital organs, are the site of the origin of the sympathetic nervous system, and are an important structural link with the upper limb. Although gross motion of the thoracic spine is limited by the presence of the ribs, physiologic and nonphysiologic motion are crucial to the respiratory, cardiovascular, and digestive organs. Trauma, postinfectious visceral adhesive pathology, and surgical intervention are possible causes of local lesions.[7] Assessment of spinal and rib motion may be useful in determining the site of clinically significant areas of fixation.

Posterior tender points may be found on the spinous processes, in the paraspinal musculature, on the transverse processes, over the rib heads, or on the posterior angles of the ribs. Anterior tender points are usually found on the anterior aspect of the sternum, over the sternocostal joints, on the anterior angles of the ribs, or on the anterolateral margins of the ribs. The tender points on the sternum are reflexly related to the anterior aspect of the thoracic spine, which is of course inaccessible to direct palpation.

As a guide to palpation, it should be noted that T2 is usually located at the level of the superior, medial angle of the scapula, T3 at the level of the spine of the scapula, and T7 at the level of the inferior border of the scapula. The eleventh rib is usually found at the level of the iliac crest.[3,14]

Clinical manifestations of thoracic dysfunction include back pain, neck pain, shoulder and arm pain, thoracic outlet syndrome, carpal tunnel-like syndrome, and respiratory and cardiovascular dysfunction. It is important to assess for and treat any significant thoracic lesions when there is upper limb involvement. In general, treatment of the thoracic spine and rib cage may be determined by postural distortion, if present. Therefore a hyperkyphotic upper back will usually be treated in flexion, and a hypokyphotic spine will usually be treated in extension.[23] The rules of priority, as determined by the scanning evaluation and by the application of the rules of treatment, will ultimately determine where and how to treat.

¶TREATMENT

Posterior lesions are treated in extension, and head and shoulder position is used to localize the release of the involved tissues at the level of the dysfunction. From appearances, it may seem, in some cases, that the area being treated is under stretch; however, review of the pertinent anatomy will clarify the rationale used. Through its myofascial connections to the rib cage, the ipsilateral arm, when elevated, causes the ribs to elevate, which in turn elevates the lower attachments of the levator costorum or multifidus toward their insertions on the lamina of the vertebrae one or two segments above.[17] Anterior lesions are treated with varying degrees of flexion with the addition of rotation or lateral flexion to fine-tune the position.

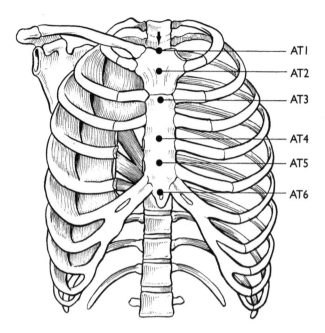

Upper Anterior Thoracic Region

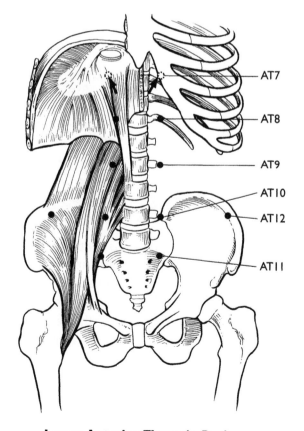

Lower Anterior Thoracic Region

THORACIC SPINE
AND RIB CAGE

40-42. Anterior First, Second, and Third Thoracic (AT1-3)
Internal Intercostal, Sternothyroid

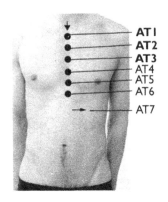

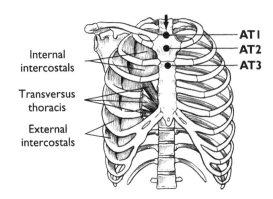

Location of Tender Point (AT1)	This tender point is located on the superior surface of the suprasternal notch. Pressure is applied inferiorly.
Location of Tender Point (AT2)	This tender point is located on the anterior surface of the manubrium. Pressure is applied posteriorly.
Location of Tender Point (AT3)	This tender point is located on the anterior surface of the sternum on or just inferior to the sternomanubrial joint. Pressure is applied posteriorly.

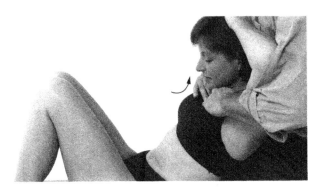

Position of Treatment	The patient sits in front of the therapist with knees flexed and hands on top of the head. A pillow may be used between the patient and therapist for comfort. The therapist places his or her arms around the patient and under the patient's axillae. The patient leans back toward the therapist, and the therapist allows the patient to slump into marked flexion down to the level of the tender point. The patient's trunk is folded over the tender point. Fine-tuning is accomplished with the addition of rotation or lateral flexion.

Note: AT1-6 may be performed in the supine or lateral recumbent positions with minor modifications.

43-45. Anterior Fourth, Fifth, and Sixth Thoracic (AT4-6)
Internal Intercostal

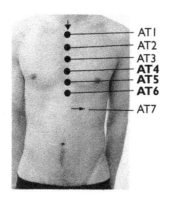

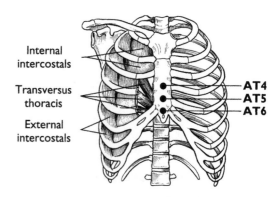

Location of Tender Point (AT4)
This tender point is located on the anterior surface of the sternum at the level of the fourth interspace. Pressure is applied posteriorly.

Location of Tender Point (AT5)
This tender point is located on the anterior surface of the sternum at the level of the fifth interspace. Pressure is applied posteriorly.

Location of Tender Point (AT6)
This tender point is located on the anterior surface of the sternum at the level of the sixth interspace. Pressure is applied posteriorly.

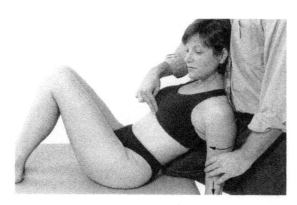

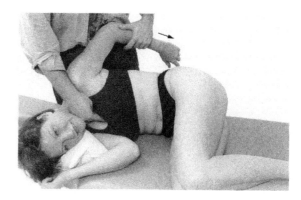

Position of Treatment
The patient is seated in front of the therapist with the knees flexed and the arms extended off the back of the table. A pillow may be used between the patient and the therapist for comfort. The patient leans back toward the therapist. The therapist places pressure on the patient's upper back to create thoracic flexion down to the level of the tender point. The flexion is progressively increased as the level of treatment proceeds caudally. Local flexion may be augmented by grasping one or both of the patient's arms and applying caudal traction and internal rotation or by having the patient clasp his or her hands behind the therapist's knee. Fine-tuning is accomplished with the addition of rotation or lateral flexion (see photo above left). The photo above right illustrates an alternate, lateral recumbent position.

THORACIC SPINE AND RIB CAGE

46-48. Anterior Seventh, Eighth, and Ninth Thoracic (AT7-9)
Diaphragm, Diaphragmatic Crura

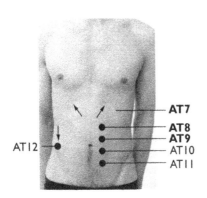
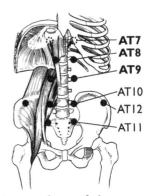

Location of Tender Point (AT7)	This tender point is located on the inferior, posterior surface of the costochondral portion of the seventh rib (pressure applied anteriorly and superiorly), approximately 1 cm (0.4 in.) inferior to the xyphoid process and 1 cm (0.4 in.) lateral to the midline. Pressure is applied posteriorly.
Location of Tender Point (AT8)	This tender point is located approximately 3 to 4 cm (1.2 to 1.6 in.) inferior to the xyphoid process and 1.5 cm (0.6 in.) lateral to the midline. Pressure is applied posteriorly.
Location of Tender Point (AT9)	This tender point is located approximately 1.5 cm (0.6 in.) superior to the umbilicus and 1.5 cm (0.6 in.) lateral to the midline. Pressure is applied posteriorly.

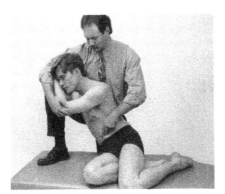

Position of Treatment Assume, for the purposes of illustration, that the tender point is on the left side. The patient sits in front of the therapist with the therapist's right foot on the table to the right side of the patient. The patient rests his or her legs on the table with the knees pointing to the right while the right arm rests on the therapist's right thigh. The therapist flexes the patient's trunk down to the level of the tender point and side bends the trunk to the left by translating it to the right. The therapist then rotates the patient's trunk to the right by having the patient bring the left arm across the body and grasp the right wrist.

Note: A physical therapy ball or chair may be used to support the arm for AT 7-9.

49-51. Anterior Tenth, Eleventh, and Twelfth Thoracic (AT10-12)   Psoas, Iliacus

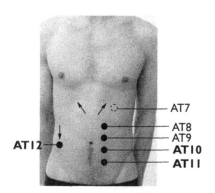

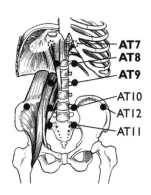

Location of Tender Point (AT10)	This tender point is located approximately 1.5 cm (0.6 in.) caudal to the umbilicus and 1.5 cm (0.6 in.) lateral to the midline. Pressure is applied posteriorly.
Location of Tender Point (AT11)	This tender point is located approximately 4 cm (1.6 in.) caudal to the umbilicus and 2 cm (0.8 in.) lateral to the midline. Pressure is applied posteriorly.
Location of Tender Point (AT12)	This tender point is located on the inner table of the crest of the ilium at the midaxillary line. Pressure is applied caudally and laterally.

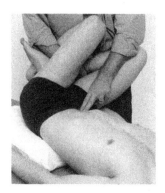

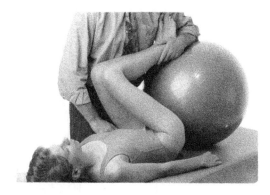

Position of Treatment   The patient is supine and the therapist stands on the tender point side. The head of the table may be raised or a pillow may be placed under the patient's pelvis. The patient's hips are markedly flexed and may be rested on the therapist's upraised thigh. The thighs are rotated toward the tender point side, and lateral flexion may be toward or away from the side of the tender point.

Note: Treatments for AT10-12 are similar, with slight variation in fine-tuning. A physical therapy ball may be used to support the legs. AT7-9 may be performed in the supine or lateral recumbent position.

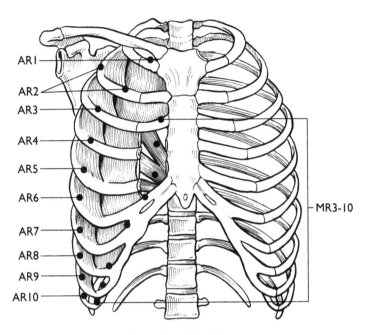

Anterior Rib Cage

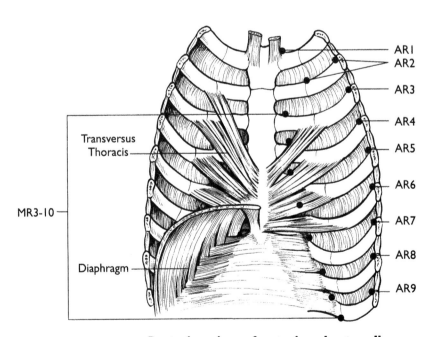

Posterior view of anterior chest wall
Relationship of tender points

52. **Anterior First Rib (AR1)**   Scalenus Anterior, Scalenus Medius

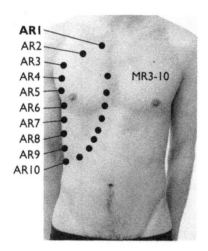

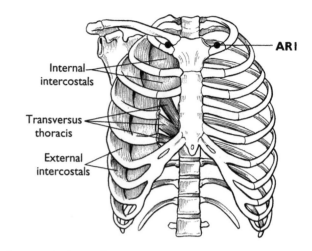

▌ **Location of**   This tender point is located on the first costal cartilage immediately inferior to the
▎ **Tender Point**   proximal head of the clavicle. Pressure is applied posteriorly.

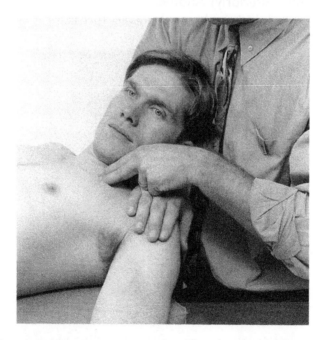

▌ **Position of**   The patient may be supine or sitting. The therapist grasps the head and places the
▎ **Treatment**   patient's neck in slight flexion, marked lateral flexion toward the tender point, and
slight rotation (usually toward the tender point) to fine-tune the position.

53. Anterior Second Rib (AR2)   Scalenus Posterior

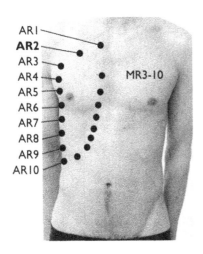

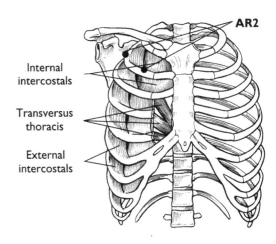

Location of Tender Point   This tender point may be found in two locations. One is on the superior surface of the second rib inferior to the clavicle on the midclavicular line (pressure is applied inferiorly and posteriorly). Another tender point may be found on the lateral aspect of the second rib high in the medial axilla (pressure is applied medially).

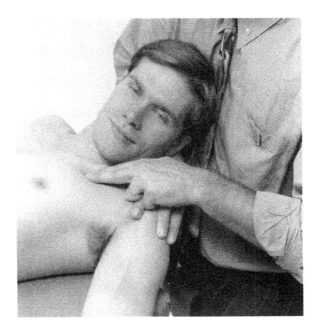

Position of Treatment   The patient may be supine or sitting. The therapist grasps the head and places the patient's neck in slight flexion, marked lateral flexion toward the tender point, and slight rotation (usually toward the tender point) to fine-tune the position.

54-61. Anterior Third through Tenth Ribs (AR3-10)
Internal Intercostal

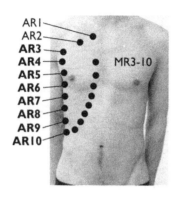

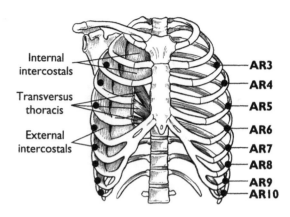

Location of Tender Point   These tender points are located on superior aspects of the ribs from the anterior axillary line to the midaxillary line at the corresponding levels for ribs 3 through 10. Pressure is applied inferiorly and posteromedially or medially.

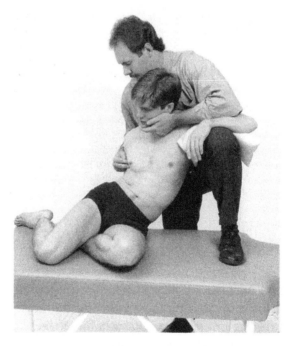

Position of Treatment   Assume, for the purposes of illustration, that the tender point is on the *right* side. The patient sits in front of the therapist with the therapist's left foot on the table to the left side of the patient. The patient rests his or her legs on the table with the knees pointing to the left while the left arm rests on the therapist's left thigh. The therapist flexes and side bends the patient's trunk to the right down to the level of the tender point by translating it to the left. The therapist then rotates the patient's trunk to the right.

Note: A physical therapy ball or chair may be used for support.

62-69. Medial Third Through Tenth Ribs (MR3-10)
Transversus Thoracis, External Intercostal

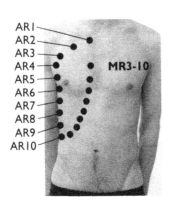

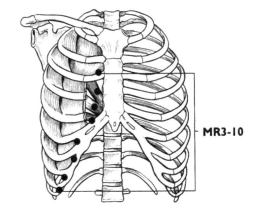

Location of Tender Point	These tender points are located on or between the costal cartilages near the sternocostal joints just lateral to the sternum at the corresponding level for each rib. Pressure is applied posteriorly.

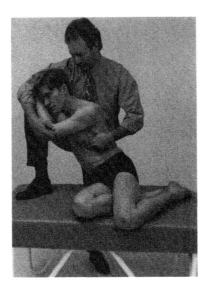

Position of Treatment	Assume, for the purpose of illustration, that the tender point is on the left side. The patient sits in front of the therapist with the therapist's right foot on the table to the right side of the patient. The patient rests his or her legs on the table with the knees pointing to the right while the right arm rests on the therapist's right thigh. The therapist flexes and side bends the patient's trunk to the left, down to the level of the tender point, by translating it to the right. The therapist then rotates the patient's trunk to the right by having the patient bring his or her left arm across the body and grasp the right wrist.

Note: A physical therapy ball or chair may be used for support.

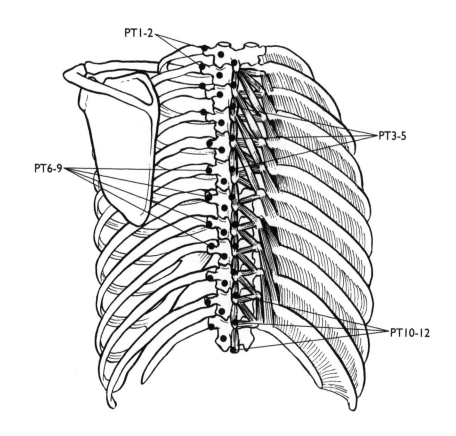

PT1-2

PT3-5

PT6-9

PT10-12

70, 71. Posterior First and Second Thoracic (PT1-2)
Interspinales, Multifidus, Rotatores

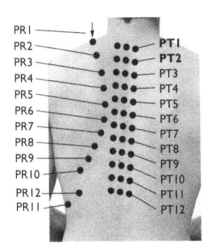

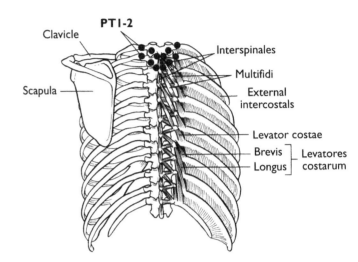

▪ **Location of Tender Point** These tender points are located on the side of the spinous process (pressure is medial), in the paraspinal area (pressure is anterior), or on the posterior aspect of the transverse processes (pressure is anterior) at the corresponding levels for each segment.

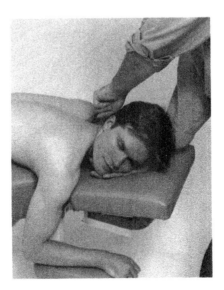

▪ **Position of Treatment** The patient lies prone with the arms alongside the trunk or abducted to 90° off the sides of the table. The therapist stands at the head of the table and supports the patient's head on the therapist's hand and forearm. The therapist extends the patient's head to the level of involvement and rotates and laterally flexes the head away from the tender point side.

Note: PT1, 2 may be treated in the supine position by extending the head off the end of the table and rotating and laterally flexing away from the tender point side.

72-74. Posterior Third, Fourth, and Fifth Thoracic (PT3-5)
Interspinales, Multifidus, Rotatores

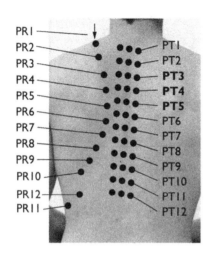

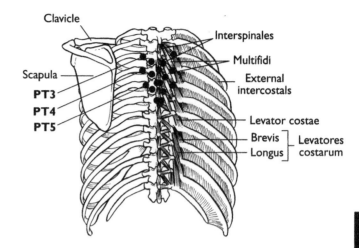

Location of Tender Point   These tender points are located on the side of the spinous process (pressure is medial), in the paraspinal area (pressure is anterior), or on the posterior aspect of the transverse processes (pressure is anterior) at the corresponding levels for each segment.

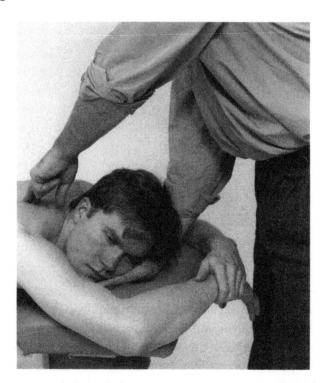

Position of Treatment   The patient lies prone with the arms on the table along the side of the head to create more spinal extension. The therapist stands at the head of the table and supports the patient's head with the therapist's hand and forearm. The therapist extends the head to the level of involvement, markedly rotates, and moderately laterally flexes the head away from the tender point side.

THORACIC SPINE AND RIB CAGE

75-78. Posterior Sixth through Ninth Thoracic (PT6-9)
Multifidus, Rotatores

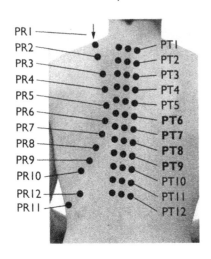

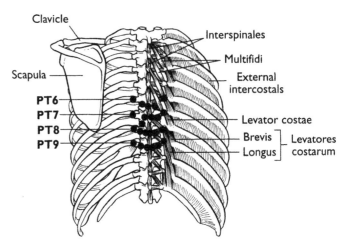

❚ Location of
❚ Tender Point   These tender points are located on the side of the spinous process (pressure is medial), in the paraspinal area (pressure is anterior), or on the posterior aspect of the transverse processes (pressure is anterior) at the corresponding levels for each segment.

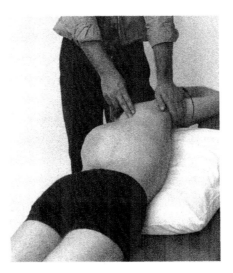

❚ Position of
❚ Treatment   The patient lies prone with a cushion under the chest and with the arm on the tender point side resting alongside the head. The opposite arm is abducted to 90° resting off the side of the table or is placed alongside the trunk. The therapist stands near the head of the table between the patient's head and shoulder on the side opposite the tender point. The therapist grasps the axilla on the affected side and pulls the shoulder posteriorly and in a cephalad direction, producing traction, extension, rotation, and lateral flexion away from the tender point side.

Note: The more lateral the tender point, the more flexion and rotation will be used.

79-81. Posterior Tenth, Eleventh, and Twelfth Thoracic (PT10-12)   Multifidus, Rotatores, Quadratus Lumborum

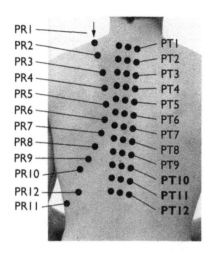

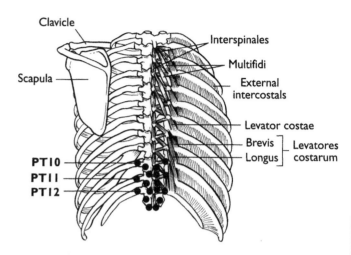

Location of Tender Point

These tender points are located on the side of the spinous process (pressure is medial), in the paraspinal area (pressure is anterior), or on the posterior aspect of the transverse processes (pressure is anterior) at the corresponding levels for each segment.

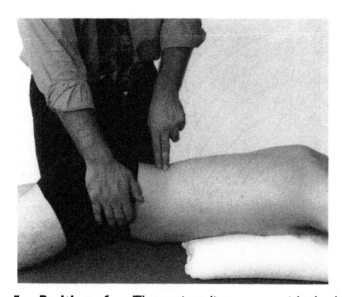

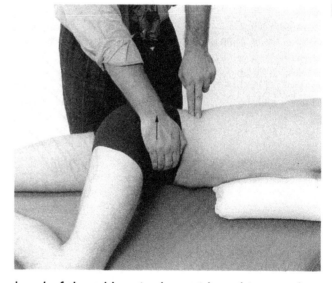

Position of Treatment

The patient lies prone with the head end of the table raised or with cushions under the patient's chest. The therapist stands at the level of the patient's pelvis opposite the tender point side. The therapist reaches across the patient and grasps the anterior ilium on the involved side and pulls posteriorly and toward the therapist, creating a rotation of the pelvis of 30° to 45°. For lateral tender points additional lateral flexion may be needed. This is accomplished by moving the patient's legs along the table away from the tender point side (see photo above left).

Alternatively, the hip on the tender point side may be abducted and flexed (see photo above right.)

THORACIC SPINE AND RIB CAGE

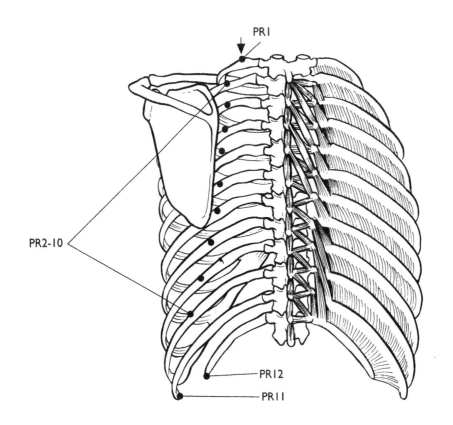

PR1

PR2-10

PR12

PR11

82. Posterior First Rib (PR1)   Scalenus Medius, Levator Costorum

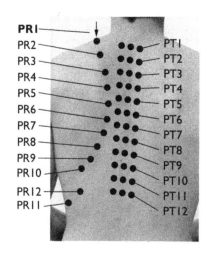

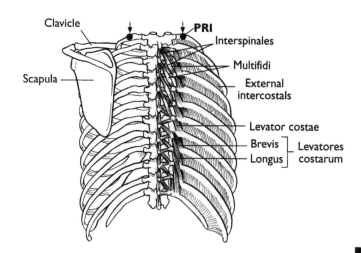

▌ **Location of Tender Point**   This tender point is located on the superior aspect of the first rib deep to the anterior margin of the upper portion of the trapezius. Pressure is applied inferiorly.

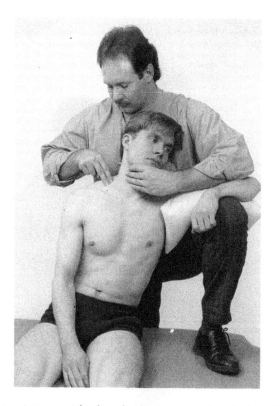

▌ **Position of Treatment**   The patient is sitting with the therapist standing behind the patient. The therapist places his or her foot on the table at the side of the patient opposite the tender point side. The patient's axilla rests on the therapist's thigh, and the therapist translates the patient's trunk away from the tender point side. The therapist supports the patient's head against the therapist's chest and places the neck in slight extension and fine-tunes the position with lateral flexion (usually away) and rotation (usually toward) the tender point side.

83-91. Posterior Second through Tenth Ribs (PR2-10)
Intercostals, Levator Costorum

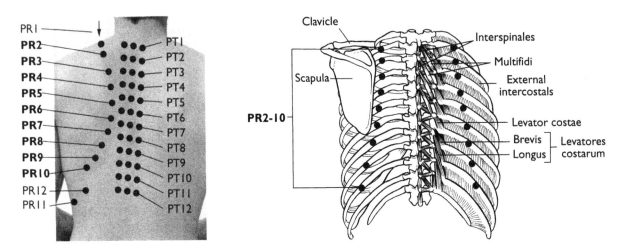

▪ Location of Tender Point	These tender points are located on the posterior angles of the ribs. To access ribs 2 through 10 it may be necessary to protract the ipsilateral scapula by adducting the involved arm across the chest. Pressure is applied anteriorly.

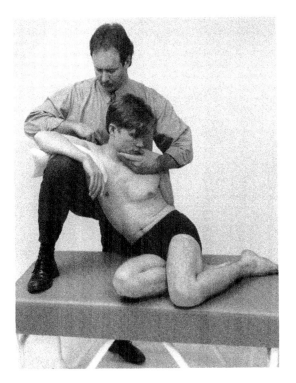

▪ Position of Treatment	Assume, for the purposes of illustration, that the tender point is on the *right* side. The patient sits in front of the therapist with the therapist's right foot on the table to the right side of the patient. The patient rests the legs on the table with the knees pointing to the right while the right arm rests on the therapist's right thigh. The therapist side bends the patient's trunk to the left by translating it to the right. The therapist then rotates the patient's trunk to the left.

92, 93. Posterior Eleventh, Twelfth Ribs (PR11,12)
Intercostal, Levator Costorum, Quadratus Lumborum

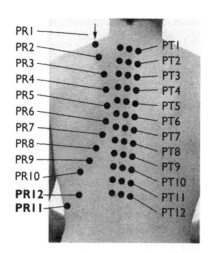

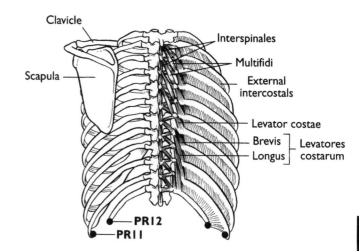

Location of Tender Point   These tender points are located on the tips of ribs 11 and 12. Pressure is applied posteriorly or medially.

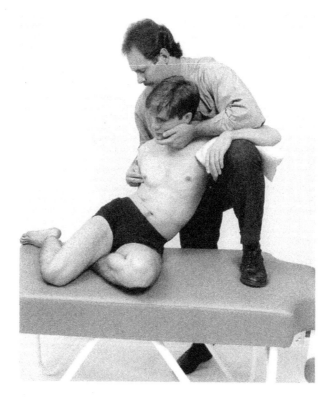

Position of Treatment   Assume, for the purposes of illustration, that the tender point is on the *right* side. The patient sits in front of the therapist with the therapist's left foot on the table to the left side of the patient. The patient rests the legs on the table with the knees pointing to the left while the left arm rests on the therapist's left thigh. The therapist flexes and side bends the patient's trunk to the right, down to the level of the tender point, by translating it to the left.

UPPER LIMB

Upper Limb Dysfunction

Pain and restriction of motion in the upper limb can arise from many sources. Local articular changes and synovial/capsular inflammatory processes can produce reflex muscular hypertonicity. Pain can originate in any of the soft tissues: joint capsules, tendons, musculotendinous regions, muscle, fascia, and even in intraosseous lesions of the long bones.[5]

The wide range of motion inherent in the upper limb afforded by the bipedal posture of the human has allowed for increased ease of manipulation and control of the environment. As in all of nature, every advantage has its price. This increased range of motion exposes us to an increased risk of trauma. The myriad uses of this versatile limb (in the quadruped its use is limited primarily to locomotion) subjects us to a variety of potential strain forces. Sudden trauma such as falls, blows, and rapid, overextended motion, as well as repetitive strain injuries, can result in reflex hypertonicity and dysfunction. This vulnerability to trauma is especially prevalent in the region of the shoulder.

Dysfunction of the upper limb is assessed on the basis of active and passive ranges of motion and strength.[10] Assuming that strength is within normal limits, restricted range of motion and the assessment of joint play affords the most precise information with respect to the specific tissues involved in the dysfunction.

Clinical presentations involving the upper limb include pain, paresthesia, weakness, restriction of motion, repetitive strain injuries, thoracic outlet symptoms, bursitis, arthritis, tendonitis, and "frozen shoulder."

With peripheral joint involvement, the tender point will often be found on the opposite side of the perceived tenderness. In general, it is advised that significant thoracic and cervical lesions be treated first according to the general rules and principles. (See Chapter 4.)

Treatment

Essentially, PRT is "applied anatomy" and treatment is directed toward reproducing the action of and shortening the involved tissues. In many cases the position is accomplished simply by folding the body over the tender point. Careful attention to the local anatomy will clarify and facilitate the position of comfort. It is strongly recommended that significant lesions of the thoracic spine and rib cage, when of equal or greater tenderness than the lesion in the upper limb, be treated first. This will greatly improve the efficiency of the treatment program. In many cases, treatment of the higher-priority thoracic lesion resolves the tender point in the upper limb.

SHOULDER *Tender Points*

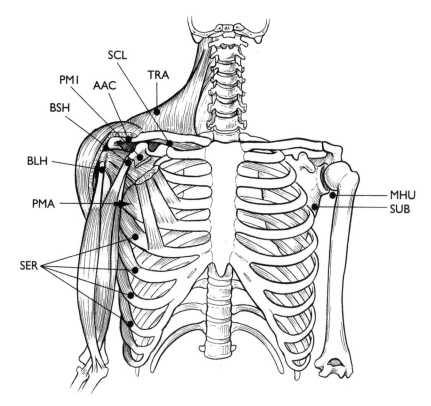

Anterior Shoulder Region

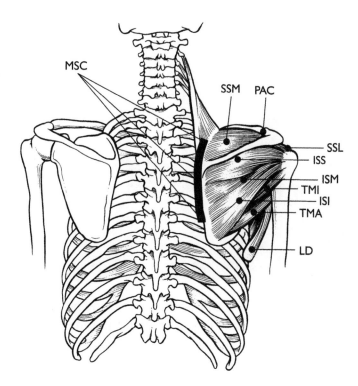

Posterior Shoulder Region

94. Trapezius (TRA)   Trapezius (Upper Fibers)

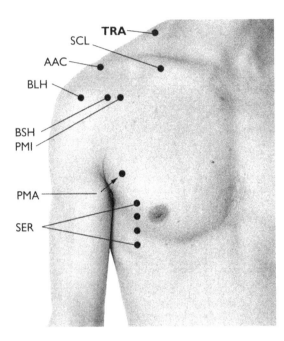

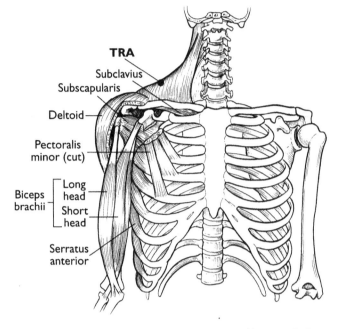

■ **Location of Tender Point**   These tender points are located along the middle portion of the upper fibers of the trapezius. Pressure is applied by pinching the muscle between the thumb and fingers.

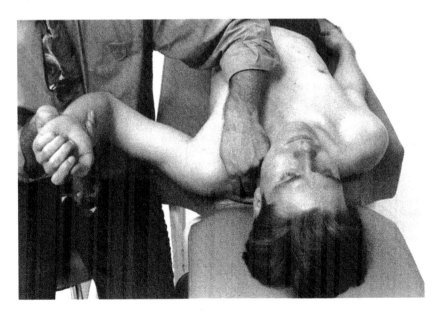

■ **Position of Treatment**   The patient is supine with the therapist standing on the side of the tender point. The patient's head is laterally flexed toward the tender point side. The therapist grasps the patient's forearm and abducts the shoulder to approximately 90° and adds slight flexion or extension to fine-tune.

95. Subclavius (SCL)

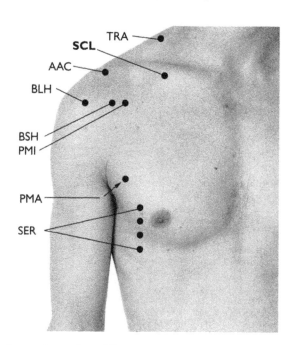

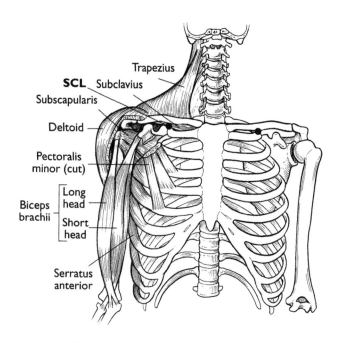

Location of Tender Point	This tender point is located on the undersurface of the middle portion of the clavicle. Pressure is applied superiorly and somewhat posteriorly.

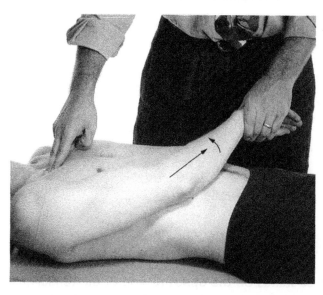

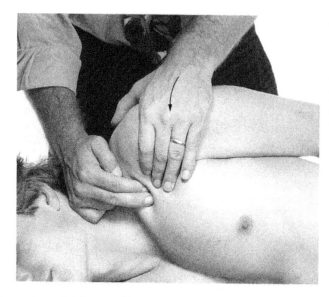

UPPER LIMB

Position of Treatment	1. The patient is supine and the therapist stands on the opposite side of the tender point. The therapist adducts the arm obliquely across the body approximately 30° and adds slight traction caudally. (See photo above left.)
	2. The patient is lateral recumbent with the tender point on the superior side. The therapist stands behind the patient and places the affected arm in slight extension behind the patient's back. Pressure is applied to the affected shoulder to cause it to be adducted in the transverse plane. Retraction or protraction and flexion or extension are added for fine-tuning. (See photo above right.)

96. Anterior Acromioclavicular (AAC)   Anterior Deltoid, Pectoralis Minor

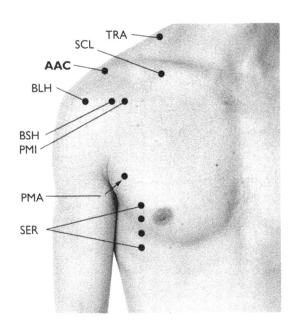

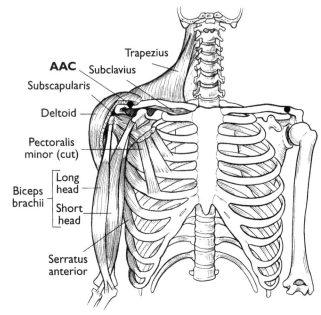

Location of Tender Point   This tender point is located on the anterior aspect of the acromioclavicular joint near the distal end of the clavicle. Pressure is applied posteriorly.

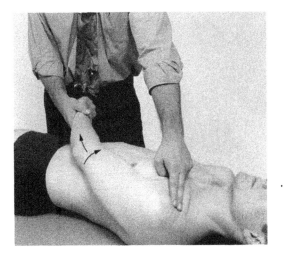

Position of Treatment

1. The patient is supine. The therapist stands on the opposite side of the tender point and grasps the patient's affected arm above the wrist. The therapist then slightly flexes and adducts the arm obliquely across the body at an angle of approximately 30° and adds a moderate amount of caudal traction in the direction of the opposite ilium.

2. The patient is supine and the therapist stands on the side of the tender point. The therapist grasps the affected forearm and flexes the arm to approximately 90° and fine-tunes with slight adduction and internal rotation.

97. Supraspinatus Lateral (SSL)   Supraspinatus Tendon

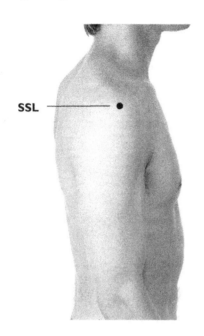

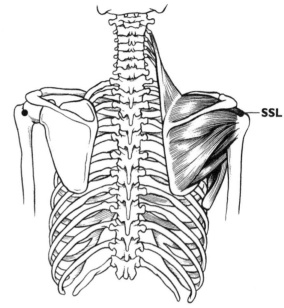

Location of Tender Point   This tender point is located deep to the belly of the lateral deltoid muscle just inferior to the acromion process. The therapist must flex or abduct the arm to approximately 90° in order to slacken the deltoid sufficiently to allow for palpation of the tender point. Pressure is applied inferiorly.

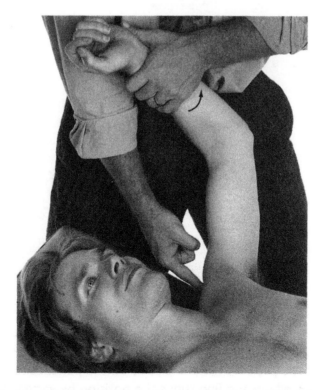

Position of Treatment   The patient is supine. The therapist produces a combination of flexion and abduction of the arm to approximately 120° and adds slight external rotation to fine-tune.

UPPER LIMB

98. Biceps Long Head (BLH)

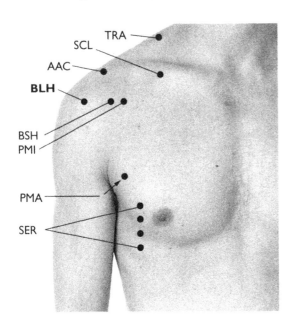

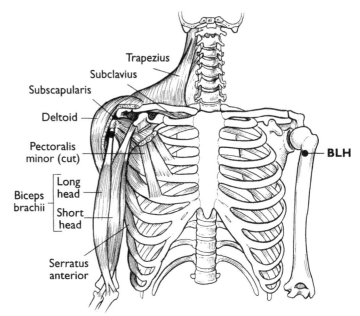

| **Location of Tender Point** | This tender point is located on the tendon of the long head of the biceps in the bicipital groove. Pressure is applied posteriorly. |

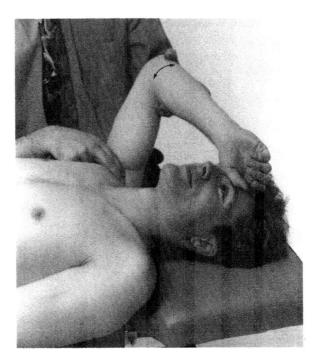

| **Position of Treatment** | The patient lies supine with the therapist standing on the side of the tender point. The therapist flexes and abducts the patient's shoulder and flexes the elbow, and the dorsum of the patient's hand is placed on the patient's forehead. The therapist grasps the patient's elbow and fine-tunes the position by varying the amount of abduction and internal or external rotation. |

99. Subscapularis (SUB)

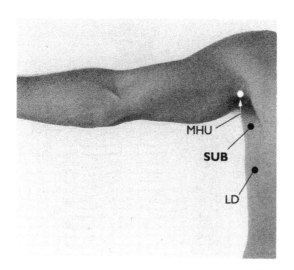

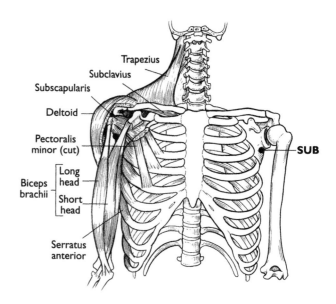

Location of Tender Point
This tender point is located on the anterior surface of the lateral border of the scapula. Pressure is applied medially and then posteriorly.

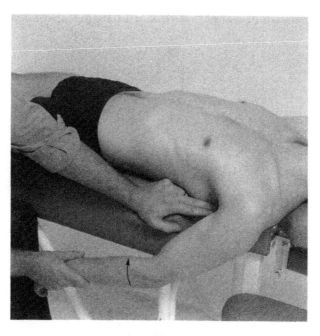

Position of Treatment
The patient is supine with the lateral aspect of the trunk on the involved side even with the edge of the table. The therapist stands or sits on the tender point side and grasps the forearm of the patient and places the shoulder in approximately 30° of extension, adduction, and internal rotation. The shoulder may be elevated to fine-tune the position.

Note: This technique can also be performed in side lying with the tender point side up.

UPPER LIMB

100. Serratus Anterior (SER)

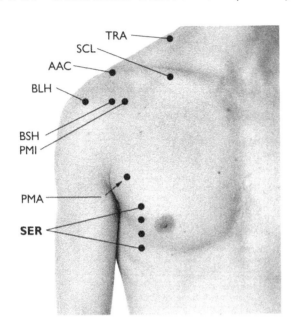
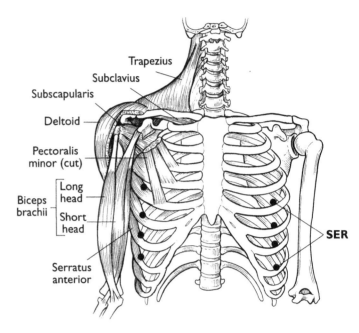

Location of Tender Point	These tender points are located on the costal attachments of the serratus anterior on the anterolateral aspects of ribs 3 through 7. Pressure is applied medially.

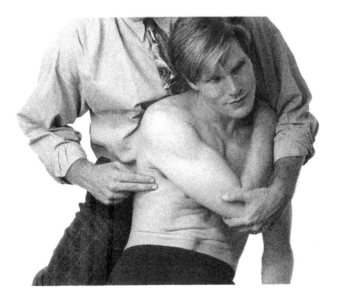

Position of Treatment	The patient is seated or supine. The therapist contacts the tender point with his or her ipsilateral hand and then grasps the involved arm anteriorly with the other hand. The arm is drawn across the chest in horizontal adduction and flexion.

Note: These tender points are located on the lateral aspect of the ribs, whereas the anterior rib tender points are located on the superior aspect of the ribs.

101. Medial Humerus (MHU)   Glenohumeral Ligaments

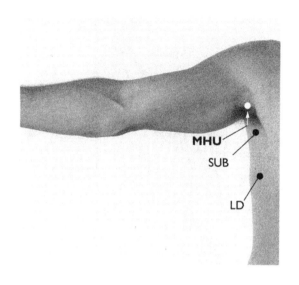

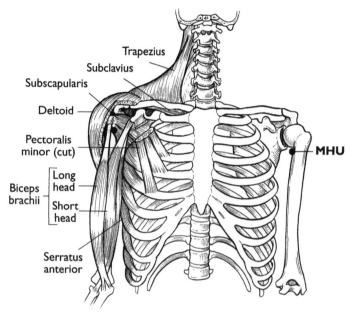

Location of Tender Point	This tender point is located high in the axilla on the medial aspect of the head of the humerus. Pressure is applied laterally.

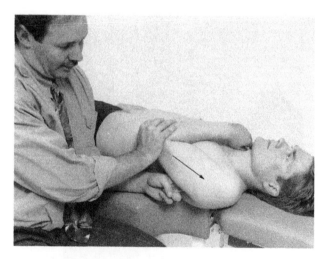

Position of Treatment	The patient is supine with the therapist standing on the side of the tender point. The therapist applies a cephalad compressive force on the elbow through the long axis of the humerus. This position results in increased adduction of the glenohumeral joint by reducing the scapulohumeral angle.

Note: This lesion may be associated with frozen shoulder.

UPPER LIMB

102. Biceps Short Head (BSH)

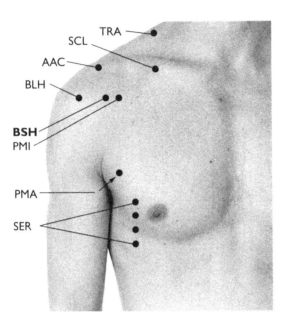

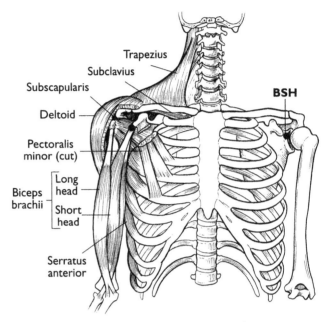

Location of Tender Point This tender point is located on the inferior lateral aspect of the coracoid process. Pressure is applied superiorly and medially.

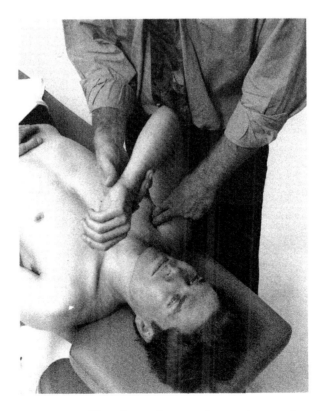

Position of Treatment The patient is supine. The therapist stands or sits on the side of the tender point, flexes the patient's shoulder to approximately 90° with the elbow flexed, and adds moderate horizontal adduction.

103. Pectoralis Major (PMA)

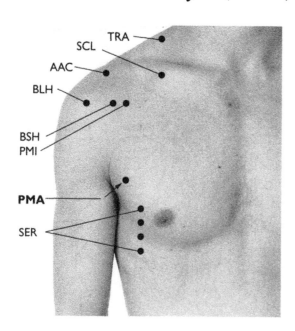

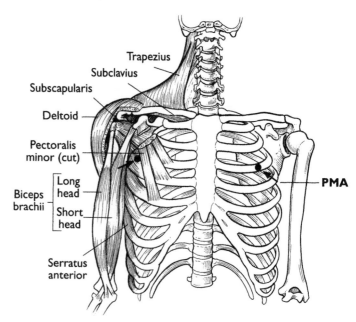

Location of Tender Point	This tender point is located along the lateral border of the pectoralis major muscle, just anterior to the anterior axillary line. Pressure is applied medially.

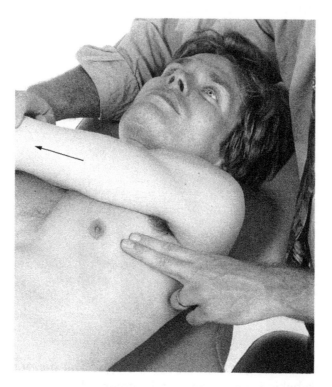

Position of Treatment	The patient may be seated or supine. The therapist stands or sits at the side of the patient on the side of the tender point. The therapist flexes and adducts the patient's involved arm across the chest and pulls the arm into hyperadduction. The therapist fine-tunes with variable flexion.

UPPER LIMB

104. Pectoralis Minor (PMI)

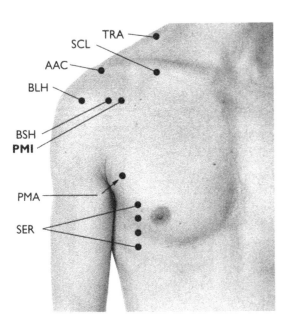

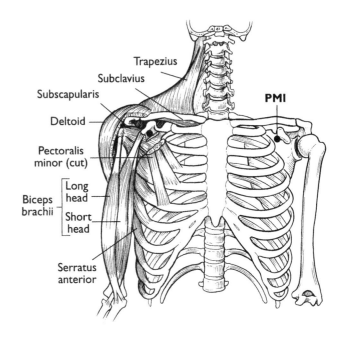

▪ **Location of Tender Point**   This tender point is located on the medial inferior aspect of the coracoid process (pressure applied superiorly and laterally) or on the anterior aspect of ribs 2, 3, and 4 just lateral to the midclavicular line (pressure applied posteriorly and medially).

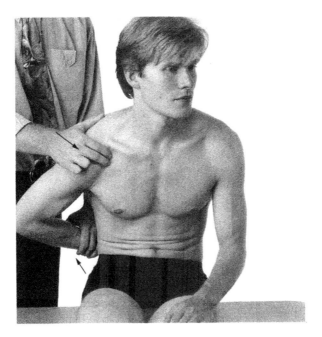

▪ **Position of Treatment**   The patient is sitting in front of the therapist. The therapist grasps the forearm and pulls it behind the patient in a hammerlock position in order to extend and internally rotate the shoulder. The therapist then protracts the shoulder by pushing the elbow or shoulder forward, abducting slightly and pushing anteriorly on the involved shoulder.

105. Latissimus Dorsi (LD)

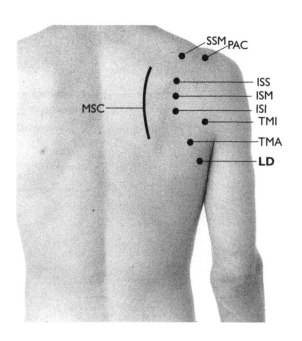

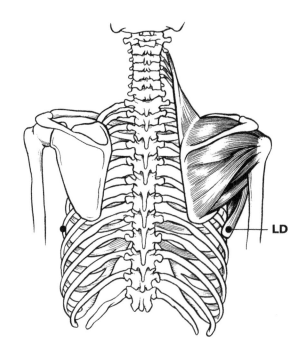

Location of Tender Point　This tender point is located on the anterior medial aspect of the humerus just medial to the bicipital groove (pressure applied posterolaterally). Another point may be found 2 to 3 cm (0.8 to 1.2 in.) lateral to inferior angle of the scapula. Pressure is applied anteriorly.

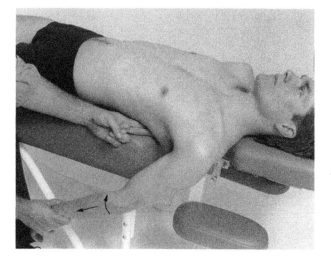

Position of Treatment　The patient is supine with the lateral aspect of the trunk on the involved side, even with the edge of the table. The therapist stands or sits on the tender point side, grasps the forearm of the patient, and places the shoulder in approximately 30° of extension, adduction, and internal rotation. Long-axis traction is then applied to the arm.

Note: This technique can also be performed in side lying with the tender point side up.

UPPER LIMB

106. Posterior Acromioclavicular (PAC)   AC Ligament

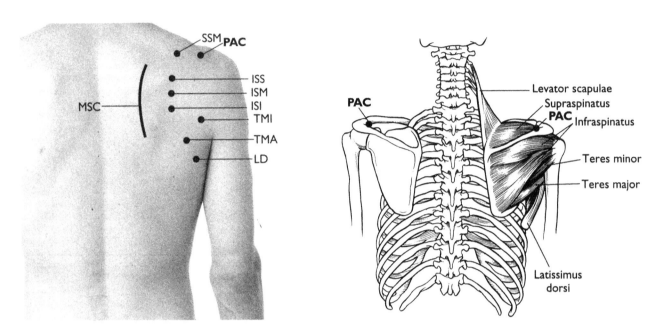

<table>
</table>

| | Location of Tender Point | This tender point is located on the posterior aspect of the acromioclavicular joint near the distal end of the clavicle. Pressure is applied anteriorly. |

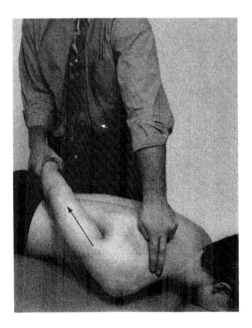

| | Position of Treatment | The patient is prone and the therapist stands on the side opposite the tender point. The therapist grasps the patient's involved arm and pulls it obliquely across the body approximately 30° and applies caudal traction toward the opposite hip. |

107. Supraspinatus Medial (SSM)   Supraspinatus Muscle

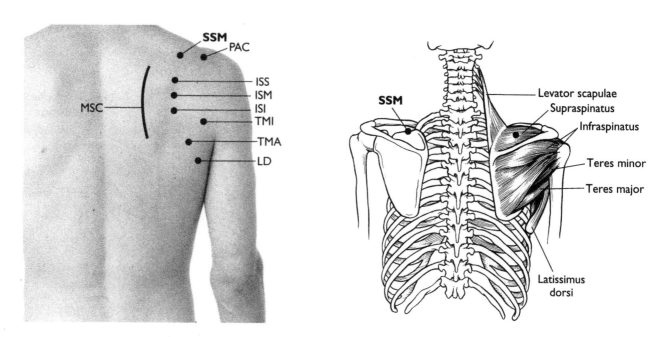

> **Location of Tender Point**
>
> This tender point is located in the belly of the supraspinatus muscle in the supraspinous fossa or at the musculotendinous junction just medial to the posterior aspect of the acromioclavicular joint. Pressure is applied anteriorly and inferiorly.

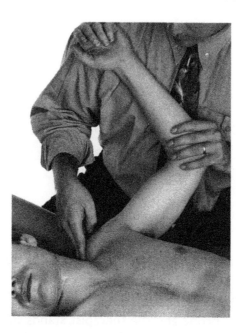

> **Position of Treatment**
>
> The patient lies supine. The therapist is on the side of the tender point. The therapist grasps the forearm near the elbow and places the shoulder into 45° of flexion, abduction, and external rotation.

UPPER LIMB

108. Medial Scapula (MSC)   Levator Scapula, Rhomboid

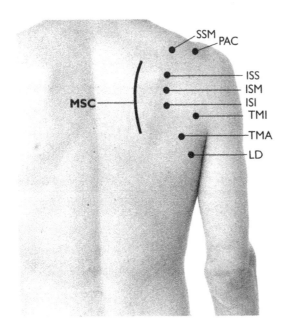

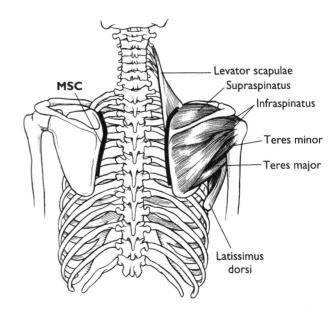

Location of Tender Point   These tender points are located on the superior vertebral angle of the scapula and along the medial border of the scapula. Pressure is applied caudally, laterally, or both.

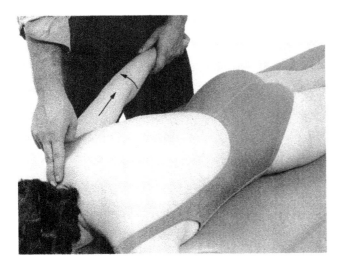

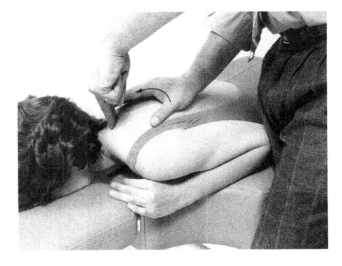

Position of Treatment

1. The patient is prone and the therapist stands on the side of the tender point. The affected arm is grasped above the wrist, extended 20° to 30°, internally rotated, and tractioned caudally.

2. The patient is prone and the therapist stands on the side of the tender point. The patient's forearm is flexed at the elbow and the hand is placed under the affected shoulder. The therapist pushes the lateral aspect of the inferior angle of the scapula medially and cephalad.

3. The patient is supine. The therapist flexes the shoulder to approximately 110° to 120° with the elbow flexed and fine-tunes the position with internal or external rotation.

109. Infraspinatus Superior (ISS)   Infraspinatus (Superior Fibers)

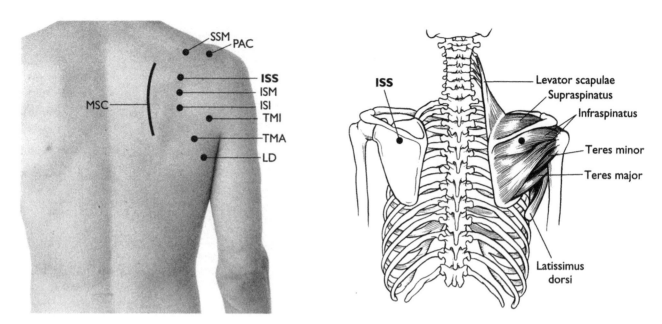

Location of Tender Point	This tender point is located along the inferior border of the spine of the scapula. Pressure is applied anteriorly.

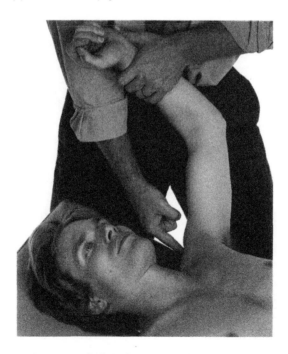

Position of Treatment	The patient is supine and the therapist is on the side of the tender point. The therapist grasps the forearm and flexes the shoulder to approximately 90° to 100° with moderate horizontal abduction and slight external rotation.
	Note: This treatment can also be done with the patient in prone with the therapist standing on the opposite side of the tender point. Place a rolled up towel under the affected shoulder. Therapist pushes the medical aspect of the inferior angle of the scapula laterally and cephalad.

UPPER LIMB

110. Infraspinatus Middle (ISM)   Infraspinatus (Middle Fibers)

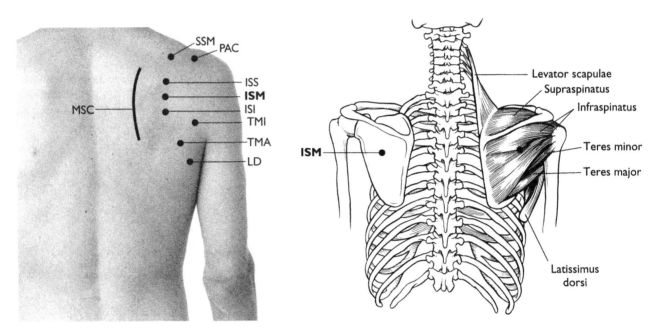

Location of Tender Point	This tender point is located in the upper portion of the infraspinous fossa. Pressure is applied anteriorly.

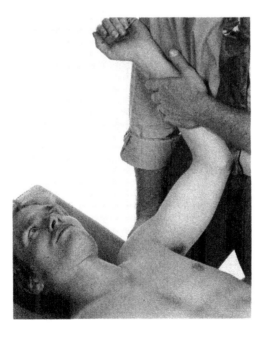

Position of Treatment	The patient is supine and the therapist stands on the side of the tender point. The therapist grasps the forearm and flexes the shoulder to approximately 110° to 120° with moderate horizontal abduction and slight external rotation.
	Note: This treatment can also be done with the patient in prone with the therapist standing on the opposite side of the tender point. Place a rolled up towel under the affected shoulder. Therapist pushes the medical aspect of the inferior angle of the scapula laterally and cephalad.

111. Infraspinatus Inferior (ISI)   Infraspinatus (Inferior Fibers)

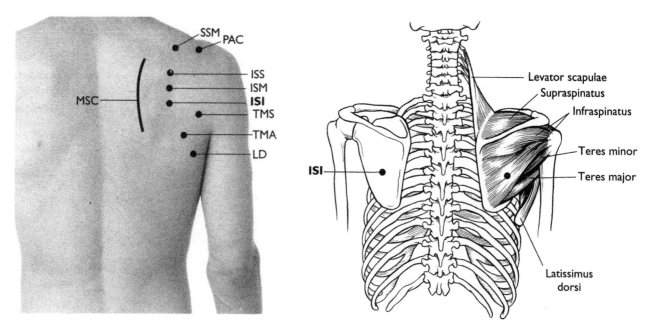

Location of Tender Point	This tender point is located in the central or lower portion of the infraspinous fossa. Pressure is applied anteriorly.

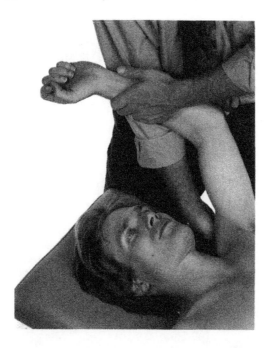

Position of Treatment	The patient is supine and the therapist stands on the side of the tender point. The therapist grasps the forearm, flexes the shoulder to approximately 130° to 140°, and fine-tunes with slight abduction/adduction and internal/external rotation.

Note: This treatment can also be done with the patient in prone with the therapist standing on the opposite side of the tender point. Place a rolled up towel under the affected shoulder. Therapist pushes the medical aspect of the inferior angle of the scapula laterally and cephalad.

112. Teres Major (TMA)

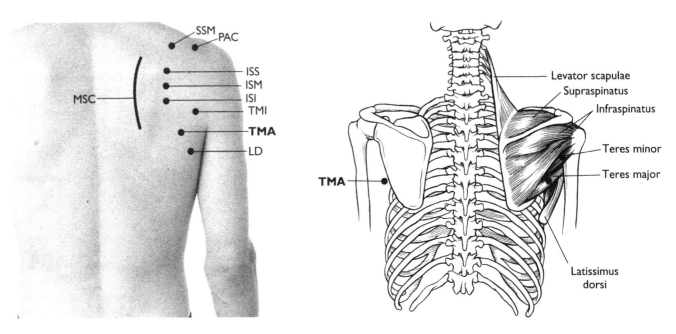

Location of Tender Point   This tender point is located along the lateral aspect of the inferior angle of the scapula. Pressure is applied anteromedially.

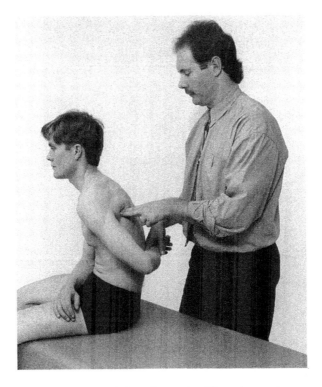

Position of Treatment   The patient sits in front of the therapist. The therapist grasps the patient's forearm, bends the arm at the elbow, and produces marked internal rotation, adduction, and slight extension (hammerlock position). Internal rotation may be augmented by pulling the forearm posteriorly.

113. Teres Minor (TMI)

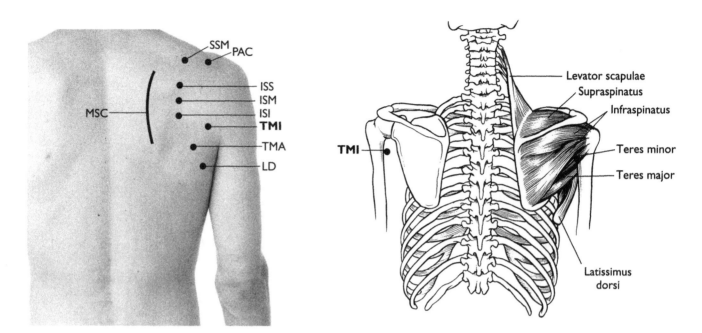

Location of Tender Point
This tender point is located on the upper third of the lateral border of the scapula or along the posterior, inferior border of the axilla. Pressure is applied anteriorly, medially, or both.

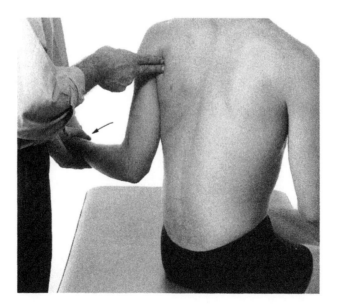

Position of Treatment
The patient sits in front of the therapist. The therapist grasps the involved forearm, which is bent at the elbow. The shoulder is extended to approximately 30°, adducted, and markedly externally rotated.

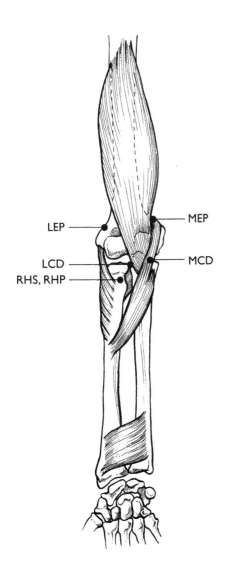

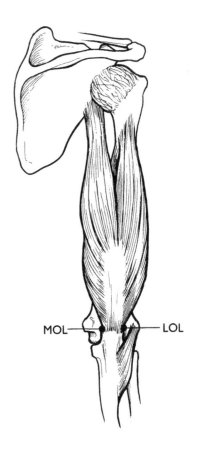

114. Lateral Epicondyle (LEP)

Location of Tender Point   This tender point is located on the supracondylar ridge superior to the lateral epicondyle. Pressure is applied medially.

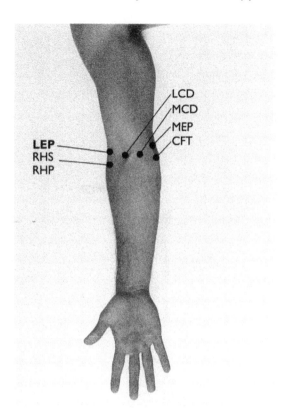

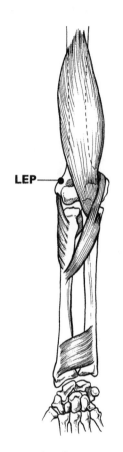

Position of Treatment   Treatment is directed to the first thoracic segment or the first rib, (AT1, PT1, AR1, PR1). Check for tender points in these areas and treat according to the general rules. Monitor the LEP tender point during and after the treatment.

115. Medial Epicondyle (MEP)

Location of Tender Point This tender point is located on the supracondylar ridge superior to the medial epicondyle. Pressure is applied laterally.

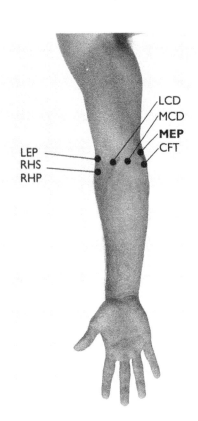

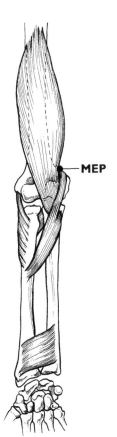

Position of Treatment Treatment is directed to the fourth thoracic segment or the fourth rib, (AT4, PT4, AR4, PR4, MR4). Check for tender points in these areas and treat according to the general rules. Monitor the MEP tender point during and after the treatment.

116. Radial Head Supinator (RHS)   Supinator

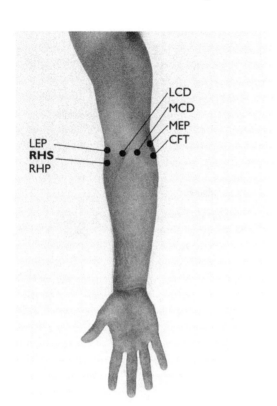

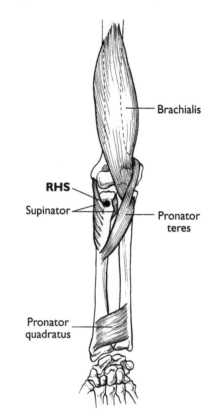

| | **Location of Tender Point** | This tender point is located on the anterior surface of the proximal head of the radius. Pressure is applied posteriorly. |

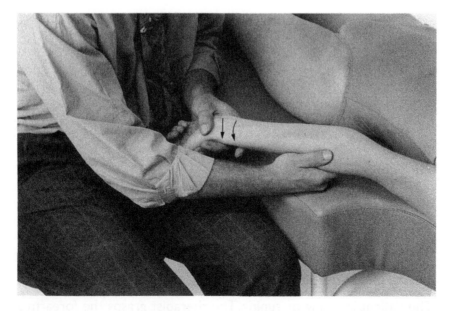

| | **Position of Treatment** | The patient may be seated or supine. The therapist grasps the patient's forearm and elbow, markedly supinates the forearm, and mildly extends the elbow. Abduction (valgus) is used to fine-tune the position. |

117. Radial Head Pronator (RHP)   Pronator Teres

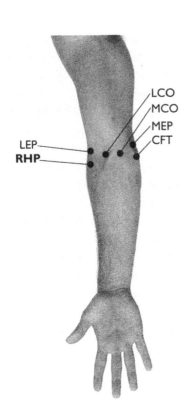

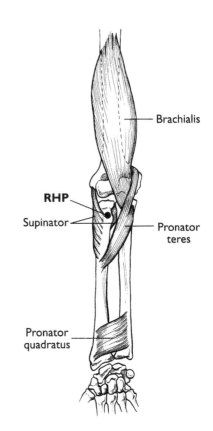

■ **Location of**   This tender point is located on the anterior surface of the proximal head of the
  Tender Point   radius. Pressure is applied posteriorly.

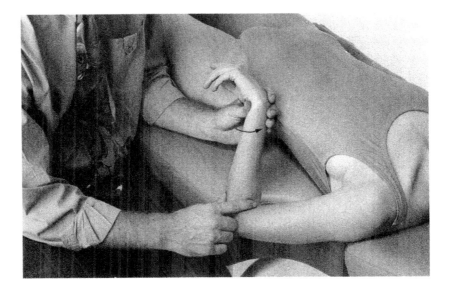

■ **Position of**   The patient is sitting or supine. The therapist grasps the forearm and elbow and pro-
  Treatment   duces marked pronation and flexion at the elbow with the dorsum of the patient's
                     hand coming to rest on the patient's lateral trunk.

118, 119. Lateral/Medial Coronoid (MCD/LCD) Brachialis

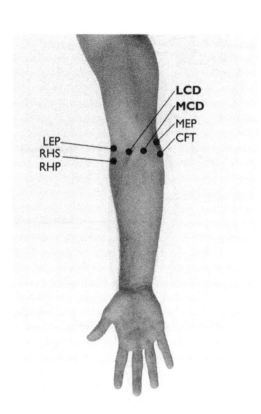

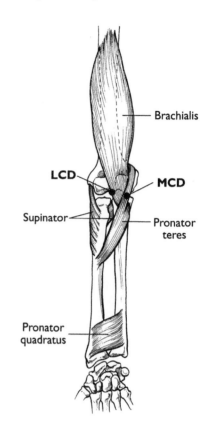

Location of Tender Point   These tender points are located on the medial and lateral aspects of the coronoid process of the ulna. Pressure is applied posteriorly.

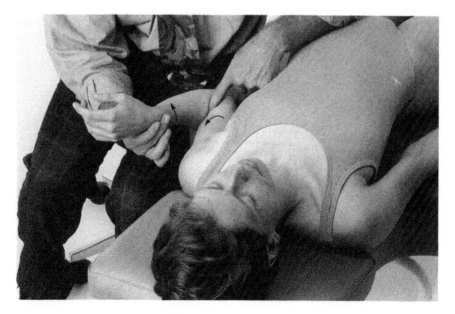

Position of Treatment   The patient is sitting or supine. The therapist markedly flexes the elbow, pronates the forearm to turn the palm forward, and externally rotates the humerus.

UPPER LIMB

120, 121. Lateral/Medial Olecranon (MOL/LOL)   Triceps

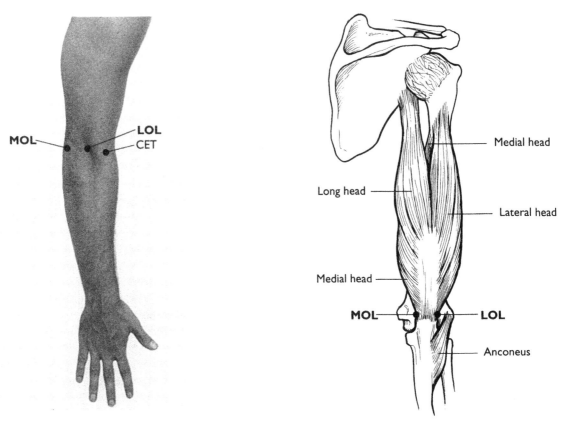

Location of Tender Point   These tender points are located on the lateral and medial aspect of the olecranon process. Pressure is applied medially or laterally.

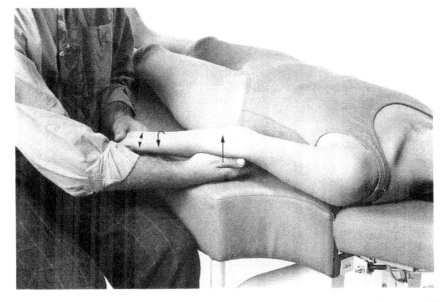

Position of Treatment   The patient is seated or supine. The therapist hyperextends and adducts (varus) or abducts (valgus) the elbow and adds slight supination to fine-tune.

WRIST AND HAND *Tender Points* _____

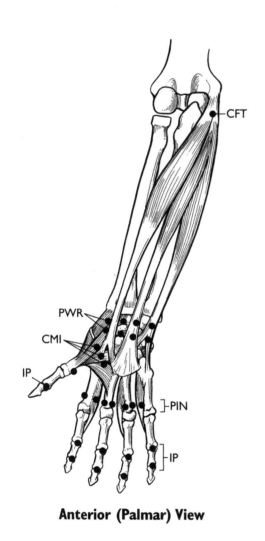

Anterior (Palmar) View

Posterior (Dorsal) View

122. Common Flexor Tendon (CFT)

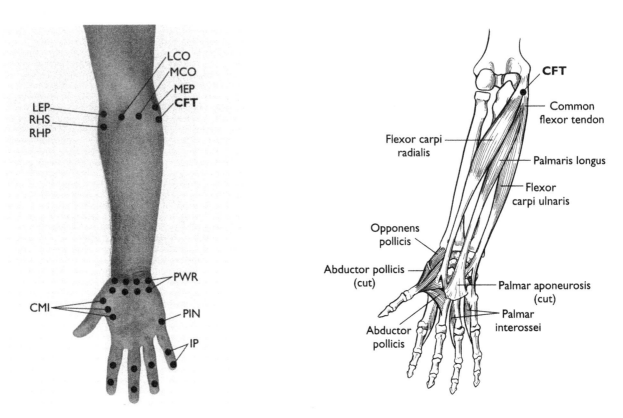

Location of Tender Point This tender point is located on the anterior medial aspect of the forearm, just distal to the medial epicondyle. Pressure is applied posterolaterally.

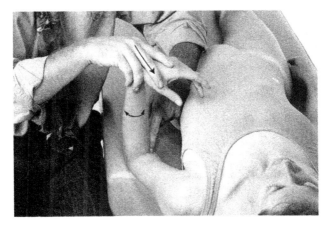

Position of Treatment The patient is supine or seated. The therapist flexes the patient's elbow and markedly palmar flexes the wrist with the greatest force being exerted on the hypothenar side. Pronation/supination and abduction/adduction are used to fine-tune the position.

123. Common Extensor Tendon (CET)

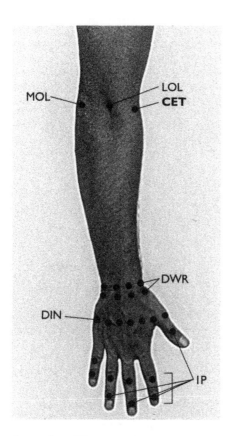

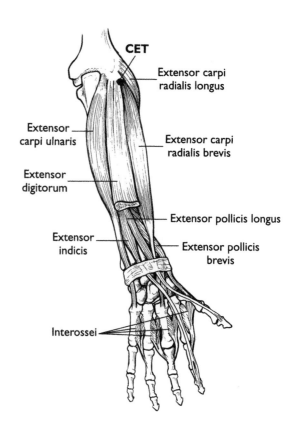

Location of Tender Point   This tender point is located on the posterior lateral aspect of the forearm, just distal to the radial head. Pressure is applied anteromedially.

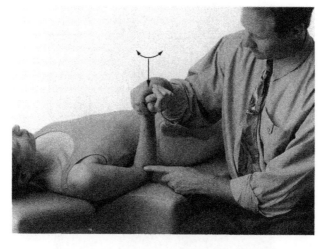

Position of Treatment   The patient is supine or seated. The therapist extends patient's elbow (not shown) and markedly extends the wrist, with the greatest force being exerted on the thenar side. Pronation/supination and abduction/adduction are used to fine-tune the position.

124. Palmar Wrist (PWR)   Wrist Flexors

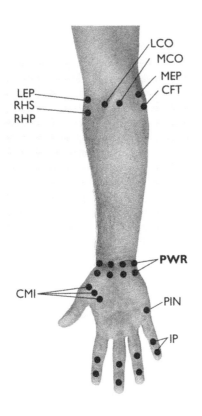

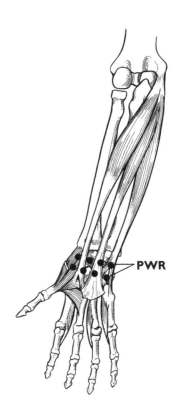

┃ **Location of**   These tender points are located along the palmar surface of the carpals. Pressure is
┃ **Tender Point**   applied posteriorly.

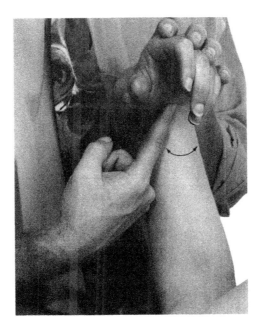

┃ **Position of**   The therapist faces the dorsum of the patient's wrist. The therapist palmar flexes the
┃ **Treatment**   wrist over the tender point. Fine-tuning is accomplished with siding, pronation or
┃   supination, and radial/ulnar deviation.

125. Dorsal Wrist (DWR)   Wrist Extensors

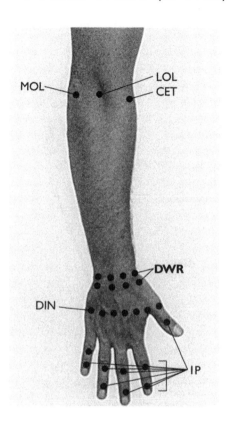

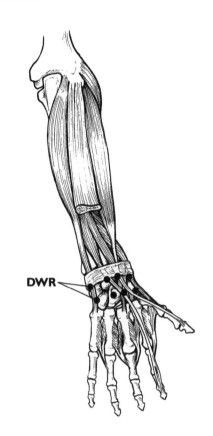

Location of Tender Point   These tender points are located along the dorsal aspect of the wrist. Pressure is applied anteriorly.

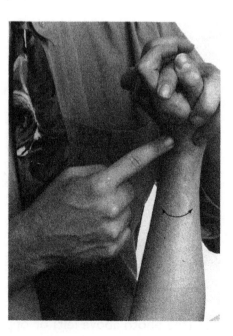

Position of Treatment   The therapist doriflexes the wrist with slight side bending toward the tender point. Fine-tuning is accomplished with pronation or supination and radial/ulnar deviation.

126. First Carpometacarpal (CM1)
Flexor Pollicis Brevis, Opponens Pollicis

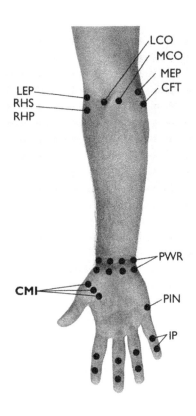

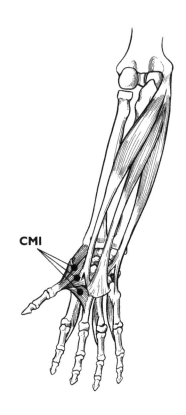

Location of Tender Point   This tender point is located in the thenar eminence on the palmar surface of the first metacarpal. Pressure is applied posterolaterally.

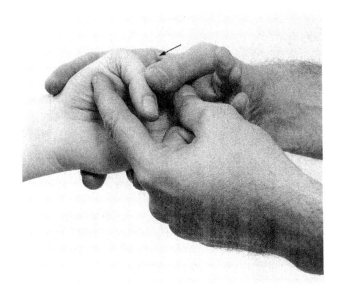

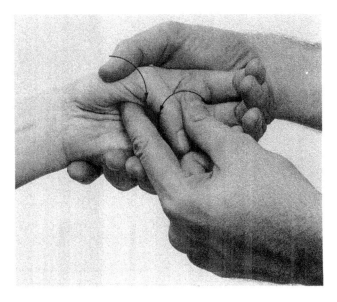

Position of Treatment   The therapist flexes (see photo above left) or opposes (see photo above right) the thumb over the tender point and fine-tunes the position with abduction/adduction and internal/external rotation.

Fingers _____

127. Palmar Interosseous (PIN)   Metacarpophalangeal Joints

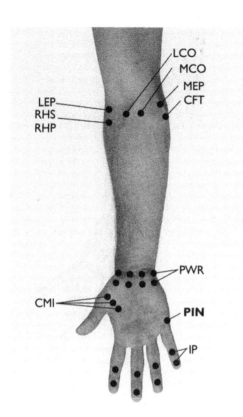 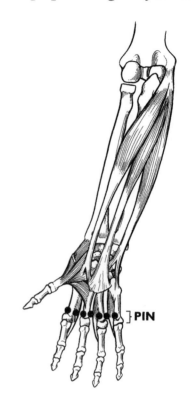

| ¶ **Location of**
Tender Point | These tender points are located within the palm of the hand, on the medial and lateral sides of the shafts of the metacarpals. Pressure is applied posteromedially or posterolaterally. |

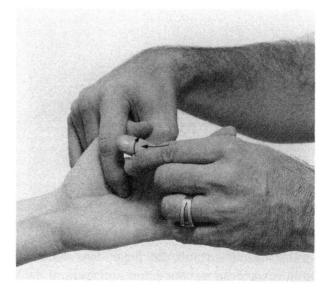

| ¶ **Position of**
Treatment | The therapist markedly flexes the fingers over the tender point with the addition of lateral flexion toward the tender point and rotation to fine-tune the position. |

Fingers _____

128. Dorsal Interosseous (DIN)   Metacarpophalangeal Joints

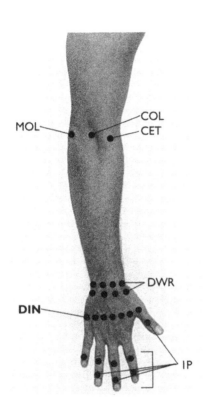

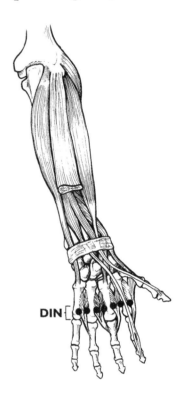

▌ **Location of**	These tender points are located on the dorsum of the hand, on the medial and lat-
Tender Point	eral sides of the shafts of the metacarpals. Pressure is applied anteromedially or
	anterolaterally.

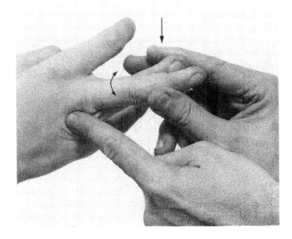

| ▌ **Position of** | The therapist markedly extends the finger over the tender point with the addition of |
| **Treatment** | lateral flexion toward the tender point and rotation to fine-tune the position. |

Note: The metacarpophalangeal joints may also be treated in a similar manner.

129. Interphalangeal Joints (IP)　Capsular Ligaments

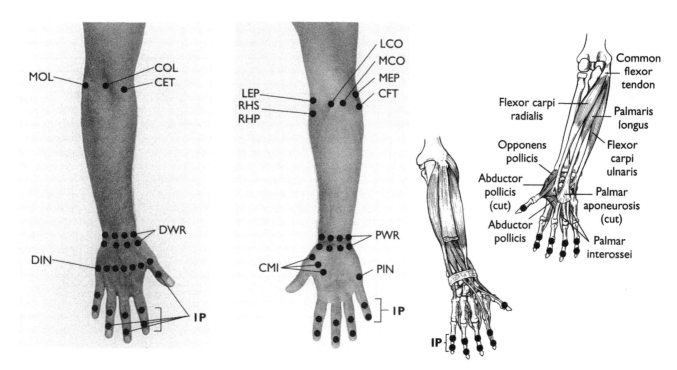

Location of Tender Point　These tender points are located on the capsule to the proximal, middle, or distal interphalangeal joints. Pressure is applied over the tender point toward the center of the finger.

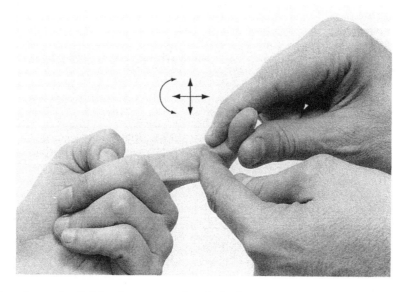

Position of Treatment　The therapist folds the more distal phalanx over the tender point, and rotation and lateral flexion are added to fine-tune the position.

Note: The metacarpophalangeal joints may also be treated in a similar manner.

UPPER LIMB

II Lower Quadrant

PRT Lower Body Evaluation

Patient's name _____ Practitioner_____

Dates   1_____   2_____   3_____   4_____   5_____

● - Extremely sensitive   ◐ - Very sensitive   ◒ - Moderately sensitive   ○ - No tenderness

\ - Right   / - Left   + - Most sensitive   ◌̇ - Treatment

XI.	Anterior Lumbar Spine (pages 144-149)				
130. AL1	○○○○○	132. AL2	○○○○○	134. AL4	○○○○○	_____	○○○○○
131. ABL2	○○○○○	133. AL3	○○○○○	135. AL5	○○○○○	_____	○○○○○

XII.	Anterior Pelvis & Hip (pages 150-158)				
136. IL	○○○○○	138. SAR	○○○○○	140. SPB	○○○○○	142. LPB	○○○○○
137. GMI	○○○○○	139. TFL	○○○○○	141. IPB	○○○○○	143. ADD	○○○○○

XIII.	Posterior Lumbar Spine (pages 159-165)				
144. PL1	○○○○○	147. PL4	○○○○○	150. PL3-I	○○○○○	153. LPL5	○○○○○
145. PL2	○○○○○	148. PL5	○○○○○	151. PL4-I	○○○○○	_____	○○○○○
146. PL3	○○○○○	149. QL	○○○○○	152. UPL5	○○○○○	_____	○○○○○

XIV.	Posterior Pelvis & Hip (pages 166-173)				
154. SSI	○○○○○	156. ISI	○○○○○	158. PRM	○○○○○	160. GME	○○○○○
155. MSI	○○○○○	157. GEM	○○○○○	159. PRL	○○○○○	161. ITB	○○○○○

XV.	Posterior Sacrum (pages 174-180)			
162. PS1	○○○○○	164. PS3	○○○○○	166. PS5	○○○○○
163. PS2	○○○○○	165. PS4	○○○○○	167. COX	○○○○○

XVI.	Knee (pages 182-192)				
168. PAT	○○○○○	171. LK	○○○○○	174. PES	○○○○○	177. POP	○○○○○
169. PTE	○○○○○	172. MH	○○○○○	175. ACL	○○○○○	_____	○○○○○
170. MK	○○○○○	173. LH	○○○○○	176. PCL	○○○○○	_____	○○○○○

XVII.	Ankle (pages 193-203)				
178. MAN	○○○○○	181. TAL	○○○○○	184. FDL	○○○○○	187. EDL	○○○○○
179. LAN	○○○○○	182. PAN	○○○○○	185. TBA	○○○○○	_____	○○○○○
180. AAN	○○○○○	183. TBP	○○○○○	186. PER	○○○○○	_____	○○○○○

XVIII.	Foot (pages 204-219)				
188. MCA	○○○○○	194. PNV	○○○○○	200. PCN3	○○○○○	206. PMT1	○○○○○
189. LCA	○○○○○	195. DCN1	○○○○○	201. DMT1	○○○○○	207. PMT2	○○○○○
190. PCA	○○○○○	196. DCN2	○○○○○	202. DMT2	○○○○○	208. PMT3	○○○○○
191. DCB	○○○○○	197. DCN3	○○○○○	203. DMT3	○○○○○	209. PMT4	○○○○○
192. PCB	○○○○○	198. PCN1	○○○○○	204. DMT4	○○○○○	210. PMT5	○○○○○
193. DNV	○○○○○	199. PCN2	○○○○○	205. DMT5	○○○○○	_____	○○○○○

LUMBAR SPINE, PELVIS, AND HIP_____

¶ LUMBAR AND PELVIC DYSFUNCTION

Low back pain is a leading cause of disability and lost productivity in our society. The lumbar spine has been the subject of extensive study and a wide range of medical interventions. Modern imaging methods are able to detect structural abnormalities with great resolution. Surgical candidates are selected much more carefully, and many surgeons recognize that the detection of significant structural pathology is no guarantee of causation or a positive surgical outcome.[2] It is gradually becoming accepted that myofascial dysfunction is the cause of the vast majority of painful conditions of the low back and that surgical procedures are inappropriate in most cases.[16]

The major focus of soft tissue therapy has been the posterior musculature of the lumbar spine. These therapies have met with some degree of success. This type of intervention often recommends the use of extension, which is also an important part of the therapeutic approach in PRT in certain cases. The diagnostic method used in PRT, however, is precise in providing direction to the use of extension *or* flexion depending on the presentation and the location of the primary tender points.

Modern humans spend the majority of their waking lives in the seated position. The effect on the lumbar flexors, over time, will be an accommodative shortening. The effect of sudden or excessive extension in the case of intermittent exertion or trauma on these shortened flexors is often magnified because of the lowered proprioceptive threshold and the contracted state of the fascia. Positional release therapy provides a powerful tool to address this common and often overlooked cause of low back pain.

Weight-bearing problems associated with abnormal function of the feet may also have an impact on the spine and pelvis. The human foot distributes weight throughout its length, from heel to toe, by way of an energy-efficient longitudinal arch. It should be noted that humans are the only animal that walks on its heels. Unfortunately, the artificial, hard, flat walking surfaces present in modern urban settings afford no support for this structure, and the deterioration of the arches of the feet may, in time, destabilize the biomechanical efficiency of the entire pelvis and spine.[20]

The pelvis is presented here along with the hip because the musculature between the two is interdependent. The pelvis has clinical significance as an important locomotion and weight-bearing mechanism and also as a housing for the pelvic viscera. It should be borne in mind that uterine, ovarian, prostate, bladder, and lower bowel dysfunction or inflammation may have an important bearing on the function of the pelvis. These organs have direct contact with the intrinsic muscles and ligaments of the pelvis, notably the levator ani and the piriformis.[6,14]

Clinical manifestations of lumbar and pelvic involvement include low back pain, scoliosis, hip and lower limb pain, bursitis, paresthesia, and numerous reflex visceral symptoms, including cystitis, irritable bowel syndrome, and dysmenorrhea.

¶ TREATMENT

Posterior lumbar tender points are located on the spinous processes, in the paraspinal area, or on the tips of the transverse processes (attachment of the quadratus lumborum). Accessory reflex tender points associated with L3, 4, and 5 are also located in the gluteal region. Posterior lesions are treated in extension, with the addition of rotation or side bending away from the side of the tender point.

Anterior lumbar tender points are found in relation to the anterior aspect of the pelvis. The tender points for the second, third, and fourth lumbar are located on the psoas as it passes over the anterior inferior iliac spine. Treatment is accomplished by varying degrees of flexion with the addition of rotation and side bending. These positions are accomplished by using the lower limbs as levers to induce lumber and pelvic movement.

Pelvis and hip tender points are located anteriorly and posteriorly on the pelvis, on the greater trochanter, or on the femur. Positioning reproduces the action of the involved muscles, and the legs are used for added leverage.

The sacral tender points were discovered by Maurice Ramirez, D.O., a brilliant osteopath whom one of us (Roth) met while both were studying with Harold Schwartz, D.O.,[18] at an osteopathic hospital in Ohio. These tender points are associated with the levator ani, and lesions are treated by simply toggling the sacrum by compressing anteriorly on an area across from the tender point. The coccyx is treated by compressing the sacral apex anteriorly and toward the tender point.[15]

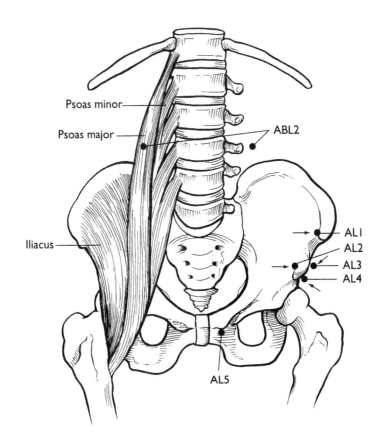

Psoas minor

Psoas major

ABL2

Iliacus

AL1
AL2
AL3
AL4

AL5

130. Anterior First Lumbar (AL1)   Iliacus

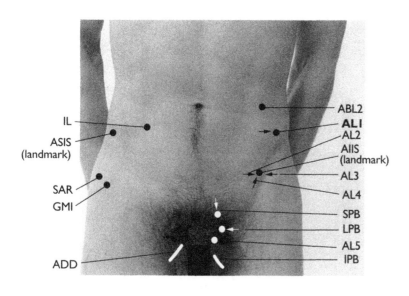

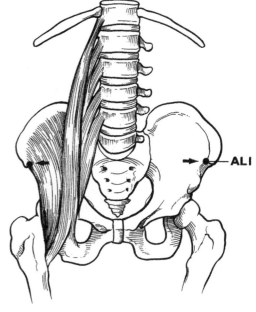

Location of	This tender point is located medial to the anterior superior iliac spine. Pressure is
Tender Point	applied posteriorly just medial to the ASIS and then laterally on the ASIS.

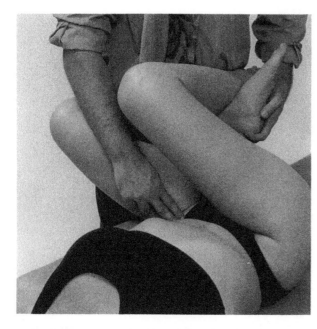

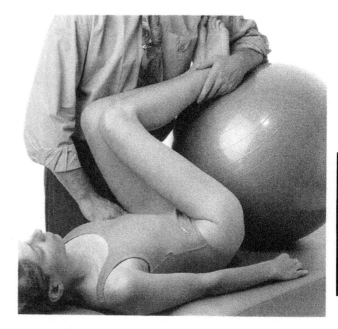

Position of	1. The patient is supine. The therapist stands on the side of the tender point. The
Treatment	patient's hips are flexed markedly, rotated to the side of the tender point, and laterally flexed toward the tender point side.
	2. The head of the table may be raised, pillows placed under the patient's pelvis, or a physical therapy ball used to support the legs to facilitate the treatment (see photo above right).

LUMBAR SPINE, PELVIS, AND HIP

145

131. Abdominal Second Lumbar (ABL2)   Psoas

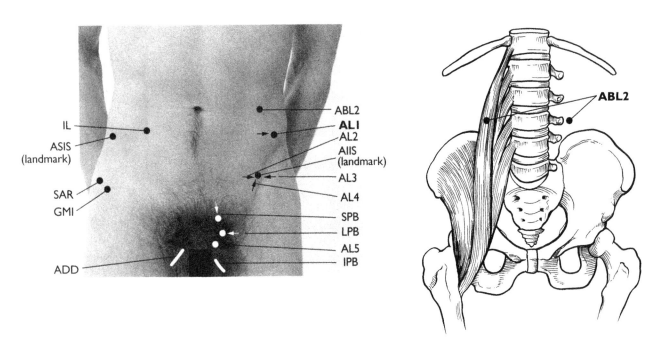

Location of Tender Point   This tender point is located in the abdominal area approximately 5 cm (2 in.) lateral and slightly inferior to the umbilicus on the lateral margin of the rectus abdominus.

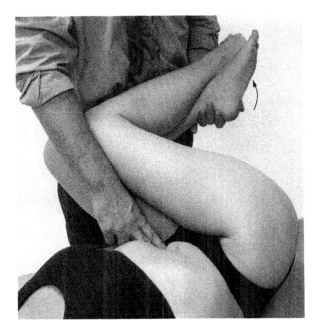

Position of Treatment   The patient is supine. The therapist stands on the side of the tender point. The therapist flexes the hips to 90° and rotates the hips approximately 60° toward the tender point side, and laterally flexes the hips away from the tender point side by elevating the feet. The head of the table may be raised, or pillows placed under the patient's pelvis.

132. Anterior Second Lumbar (AL2)　Iliopsoas

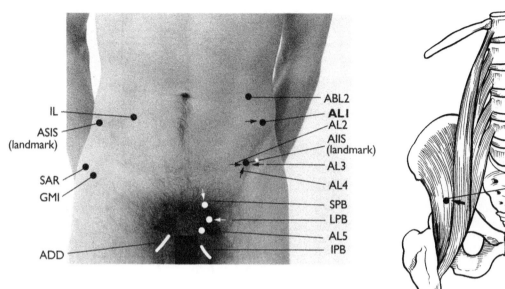

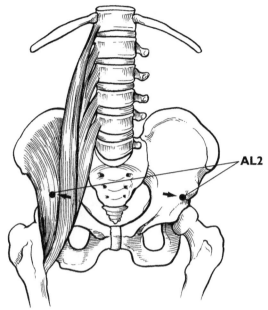

Location of Tender Point　This tender point is located on the medial surface of the anterior inferior iliac spine. The hips may be flexed 45° to facilitate location of the point. Pressure is applied posteriorly just medial to the AIIS, then laterally on the bone.

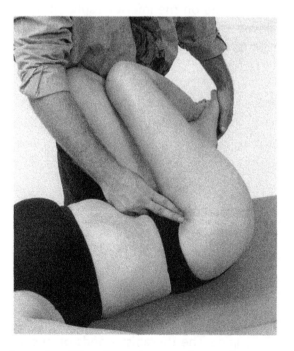

Position of Treatment　The patient is supine. The therapist stands on the opposite side of the tender point. The therapist flexes the patient's hips to approximately 90°, rotates the hips approximately 60° away from the tender point side, and allows the feet to drop toward the floor to produce lateral flexion away from the tender point side. The head of the table may be raised, or pillows placed under the patient's pelvis.

LUMBAR SPINE, PELVIS, AND HIP

133, 134. Anterior Third and Fourth Lumbar (AL3,4)   Iliopsoas

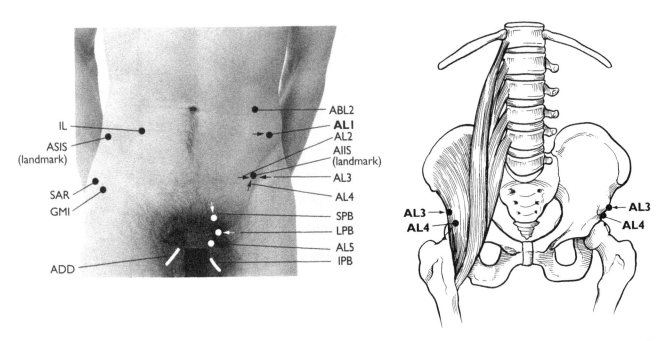

■ Location of Tender Point

The tender point for AL3 is located on the lateral aspect of the anterior inferior iliac spine. The hips may be flexed 45° to facilitate location of the point. Pressure is applied posteriorly just lateral to the AIIS, then medially on the bone. The tender point for AL4 is located on the inferior aspect of the anterior inferior iliac spine. The hips may be flexed 45° to facilitate location of the point. Pressure is applied posteriorly just inferior to the AIIS, then superiorly on the bone.

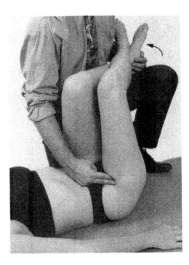

■ Position of Treatment

The patient lies supine. The therapist stands on the side opposite the tender point. The therapist flexes the patient's hips to approximately 70° to 90° and rests the patient's legs on the therapist' thighs or on a physical therapy ball. The hips are laterally flexed away from the tender point side by pulling the legs toward the therapist. Fine-tuning is added by slightly rotating the hips toward or away from the tender point side.

135. Anterior Fifth Lumbar (AL5)*   Iliopsoas

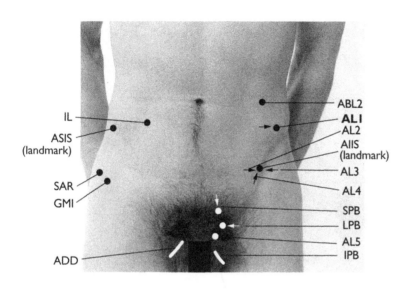

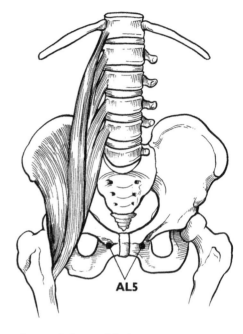

Location of Tender Point   This tender point is located on the anterior surface of the pubic bone approximately 1.5 cm (0.6 in.) lateral to the symphysis pubis. Pressure is applied posteriorly.

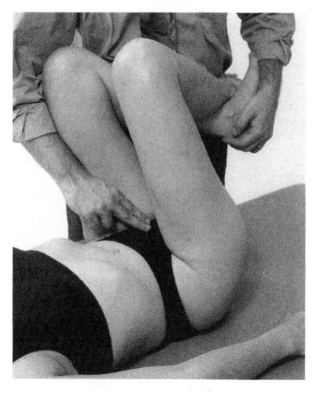

Position of Treatment   The patient lies supine with the therapist standing on the side of the tender point. The therapist flexes the hips to approximately 90° to 120° and rotates the hips toward and laterally flexed away from the tender point side.

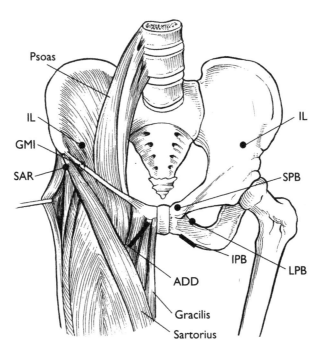

Anterior View

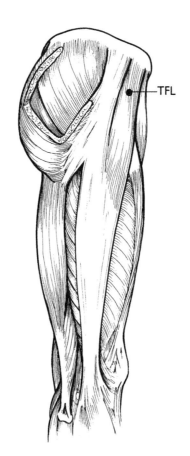

Lateral View

136. Iliacus (IL)

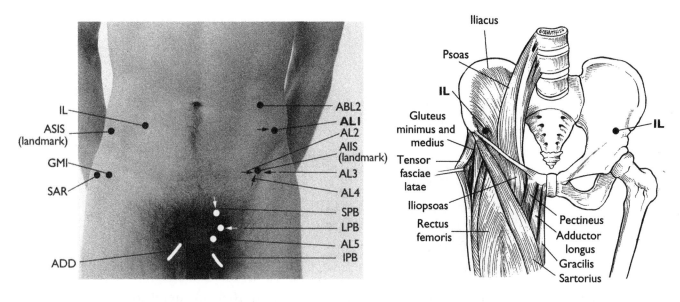

Location of Tender Point

This tender point is located approximately 3 cm (1.2 in.) medial to the ASIS and deep in the iliac fossa. Pressure is applied posteriorly and laterally.

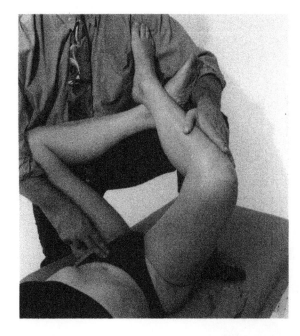
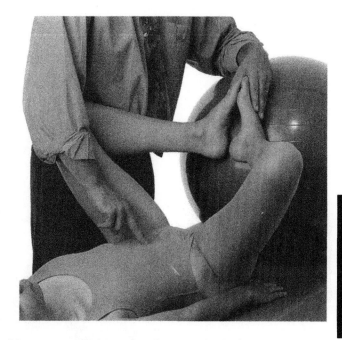

Position of Treatment

The patient lies supine with the ankles supported on the therapist's thighs (see photo above left) or on a physical therapy ball (see photo above right) or chair. The therapist stands on the tender point side and produces extreme flexion and external rotation of both hips. Rotation toward the tender point side may be added to fine-tune.

LUMBAR SPINE, PELVIS, AND HIP

137. Gluteus Minimus (GMI)   Gluteus Minimus (Anterior Fibers)

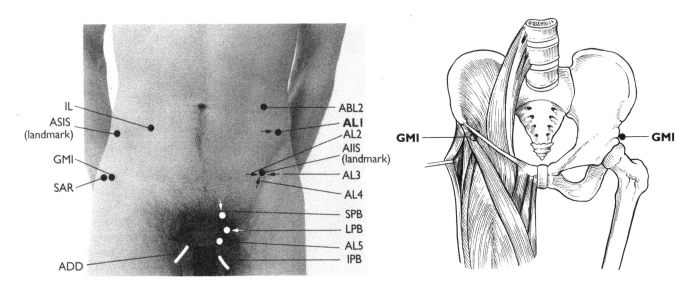

▌ **Location of**
▏ **Tender Point**   This tender point is located approximately 1 cm (0.4 in.) lateral to the anterior inferior iliac spine. The hips may be flexed 45° to facilitate location of the point. Pressure is applied posteriorly.

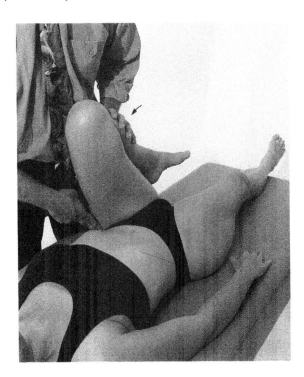

▌ **Position of**
▏ **Treatment**   The patient is supine. The therapist stands on the side of the tender point. The therapist flexes the hip markedly (approximately 130°) with no abduction or rotation.

138. Sartorius (SAR)

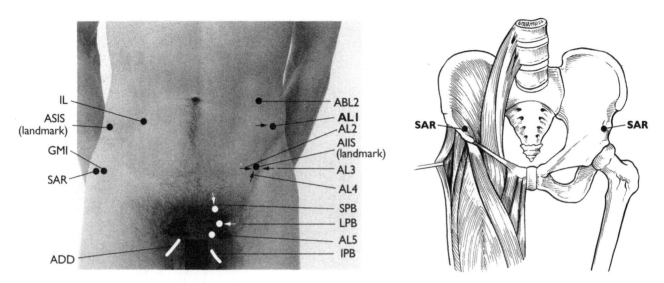

Location of Tender Point	This tender point is located approximately 2 cm (0.8 in.) lateral to the AIIS. The hips may be flexed 45° to facilitate location of the point. Pressure is applied posteriorly.

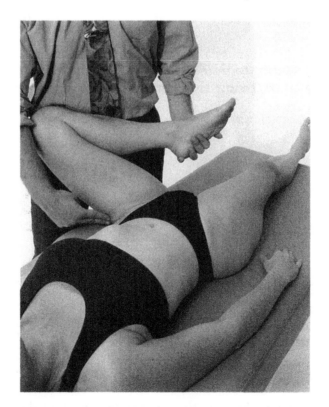

Position of Treatment	The patient is supine with the therapist standing on the side of the tender point. The therapist flexes the hip to 90° and adds moderate abduction and external rotation.

LUMBAR SPINE, PELVIS, AND HIP

139. Tensor Fascia Lata (TFL)

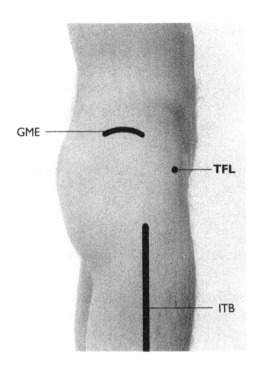
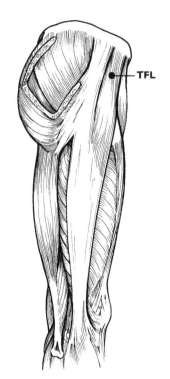

Location of Tender Point	Lateral and inferior to the ASIS and superior to the greater trochanter, on the anterior border of the tensor fascia lata. Pressure is applied posteriorly and medially.

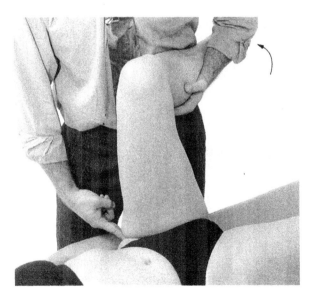

Position of Treatment	The patient lies supine. The therapist stands on the side of the tender point. The therapist then flexes the hip to 90° and adds moderate abduction and marked internal rotation by pulling the ipsilateral foot laterally.

140. Superior Pubis (SPB)   Pubococcygeus

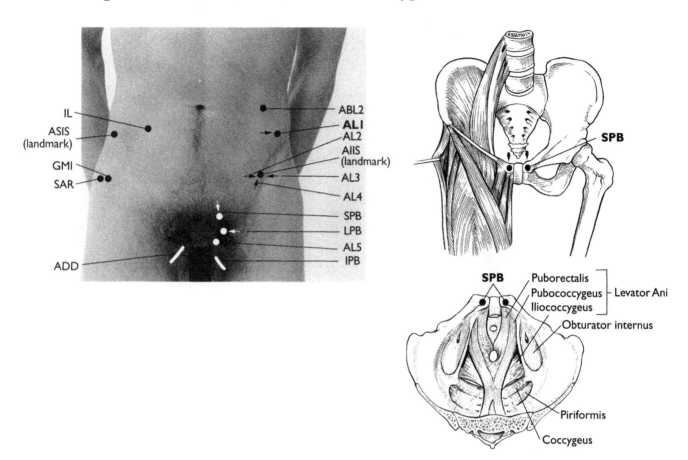

IL		ABL2
ASIS (landmark)		ALI
		AL2
GMI		AIIS (landmark)
SAR		AL3
		AL4
		SPB
		LPB
		AL5
ADD		IPB

SPB   Puborectalis
Pubococcygeus — Levator Ani
Iliococcygeus
Obturator internus
Piriformis
Coccygeus

Location of Tender Point This tender point is located on the superior aspect of the lateral ramus of the pubis approximately 2 cm (0.8 in.) lateral to the pubic symphysis. Pressure is applied posteriorly above the pubic bone and then inferiorly.

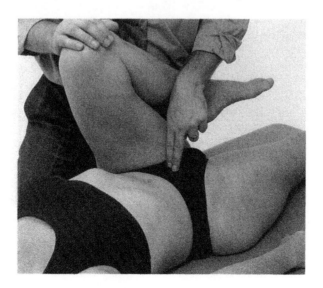

Position of Treatment The patient is supine, with the therapist standing on the same side as the tender point. The therapist flexes the hip to 90° to 120° with no abduction or rotation.

141. Inferior Pubis (IPB)   Iliococcygeus

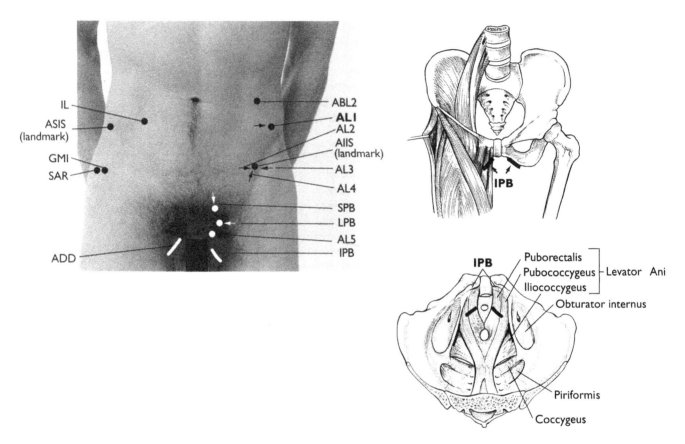

Location of Tender Point   This tender point is located on the medial surface of the descending ramus of the pubis. Pressure is applied superiorly and laterally.

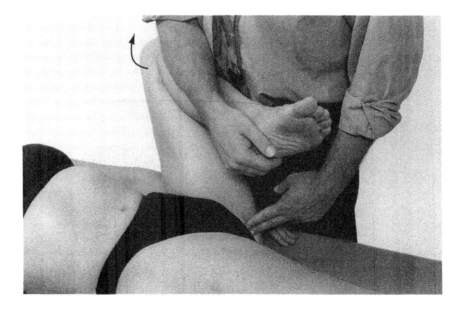

Position of Treatment   The patient is supine, and the therapist stands on the tender point side. The therapist flexes, abducts, and externally rotates the affected hip.

142. Lateral Pubis (LPB)   Obturator Externus, Pectineus

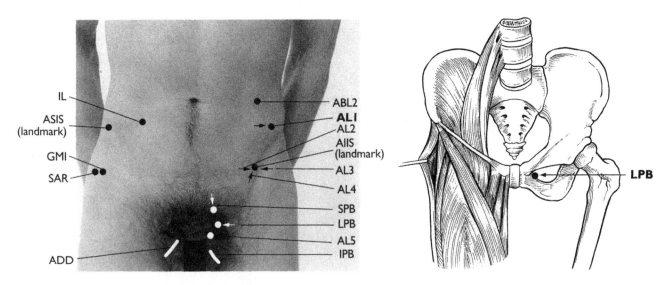

Location of Tender Point   This tender point is located on the lateral surface of the body of the pubic bone on the medial margin of the obturator foramen. Pressure is applied medially.

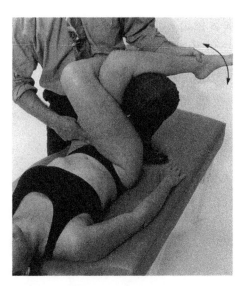

Position of Treatment   The patient is supine. The therapist stands on the same side as the tender point and flexes the patient's hips to approximately 90°. The therapist places his or her foot on the table and rests the patient's legs on the therapist's thigh. The unaffected leg is crossed over the affected leg. The therapist then uses the affected leg to internally or externally rotate the femur.

Note: A physical therapy ball or a chair may be used to support the patient's legs.

143. Adductors (ADD)

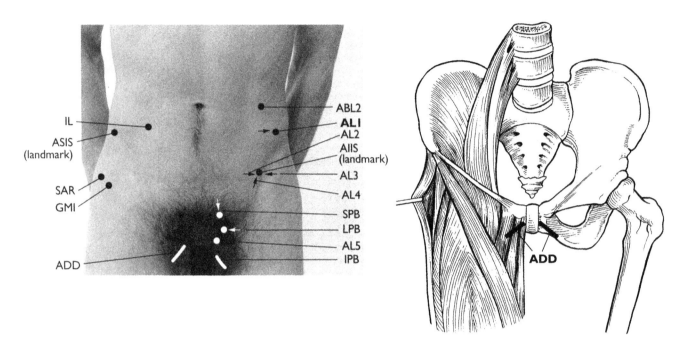

Location of Tender Point	This tender point is located on the anterolateral margin of the pubic bone and the descending ramus of the pubis (pressure applied posteromedially) or on the lower third of the adductor muscle belly on the medial aspect of the thigh (not shown).

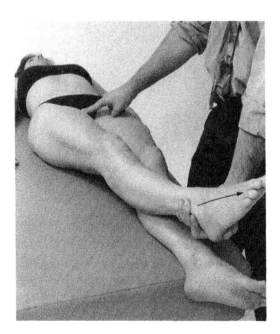

Position of Treatment	The patient is supine with the therapist standing on the side opposite the tender point. The therapist reaches across the patient and grasps the patient's distal tibia (extended knee) or the lateral aspect of the involved knee (flexed knee) and adducts it by pulling the leg medially.

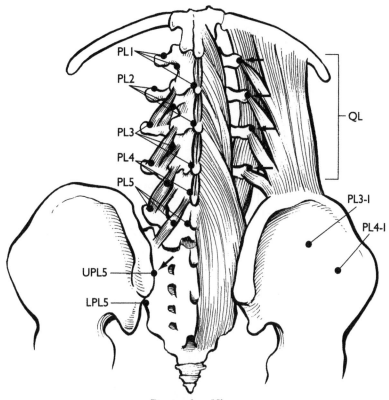

PL1

PL2

PL3

PL4

PL5

QL

PL3-1

PL4-1

UPL5

LPL5

Posterior View

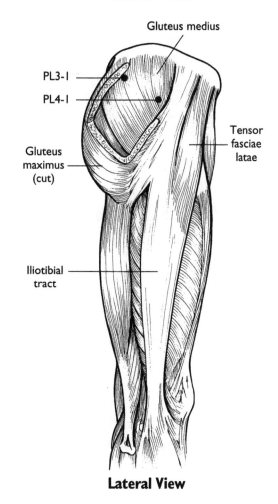

Gluteus medius

PL3-1

PL4-1

Gluteus
maximus
(cut)

Tensor
fasciae
latae

Iliotibial
tract

Lateral View

**LUMBAR SPINE,
PELVIS, AND HIP**

144-148. Posterior Lumbar (PL1-5)
Interspinales, Rotatores, Multifidus

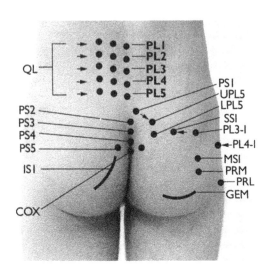

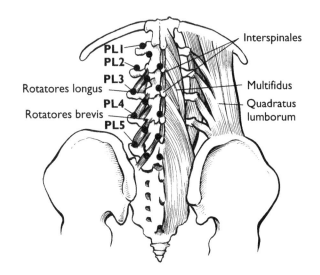

Location of Tender Point — These tender points are located on the lateral aspect of the spinous processes (pressure applied medially), in the paraspinal sulcus or on the posterior aspect of the transverse processes (pressure applied anteriorly).

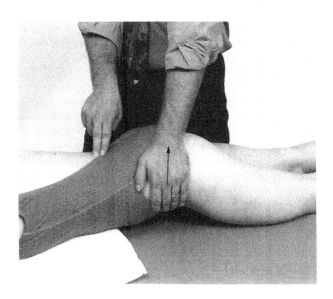

Position of Treatment — The patient lies prone. The head of the table is raised, or pillows are placed under the patient's chest. The therapist stands on the side opposite the tender point. The therapist grasps the anterior aspect of the pelvis on the tender point side and pulls it posteriorly to create rotation of the pelvis of approximately 30 to 45°.

Note: Tender points closer to the midline of the body are treated with more pure extension; lateral tender points are treated with the addition of more lateral flexion and rotation.

149. Quadratus Lumborum (QL)

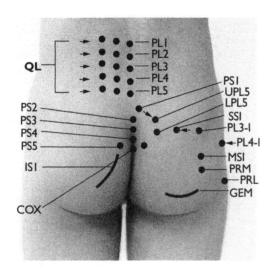

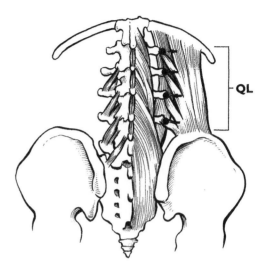

■ **Location of Tender Point**   These tender points are located on the lateral aspect of the transverse processes from L1 to L5. Pressure is applied anteriorly and then medially.

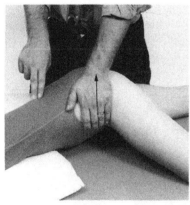
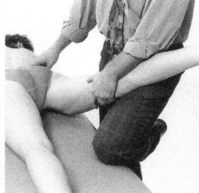
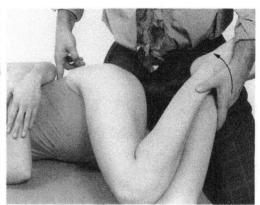

■ **Position of Treatment**

1. The patient is prone with the head of the table raised or a pillow placed under the patient's chest. The therapist stands on the side opposite the tender point and reaches across to grasp the ilium of the affected side. The therapist then instructs the patient to flex and abduct the ipsilateral hip to approximately 45° (see photo above left).

2. The patient is prone with the trunk laterally flexed toward the tender point side. The therapist stands on the side of the tender point. The therapist places his or her knee on the table and rests the patient's affected leg on the therapist's thigh. The patient's hip is extended and abducted, and slight rotation is used to fine-tune (see photo above center).

3. The patient is lateral recumbent on the unaffected side with the hips and knees flexed to approximately 90°. The therapist stands behind the patient and grasps the ankles and lifts them to induce moderate side bending of the torso. The patient's shoulder on the affected side is protracted or retracted to fine-tune (see photo above right).

150. Posterior Third Lumbar, Iliac (PL3-I)*   Multifidus, Rotatores

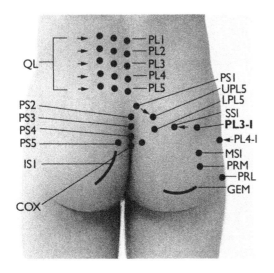

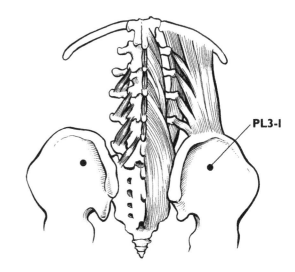

Location of Tender Point   This tender point is located approximately 3 cm (1.2 in.) below the crest of the ilium and 7 cm (2.8 in.) lateral to the posterior superior iliac spine. Pressure is applied anteriorly and medially.

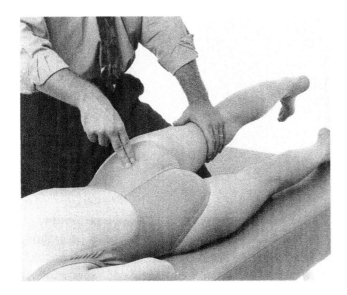

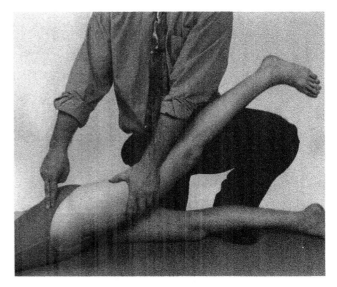

Position of Treatment   The patient lies prone while the therapist stands on the same side (see photo above left) or the opposite side (see photo above right) of the tender point. The therapist then extends the thigh on the affected side and supports it with the therapist's leg or a pillow. The therapist then moderately adducts and markedly externally rotates the thigh.

151. Posterior Fourth Lumbar, Iliac (PL4-I)*
Multifidus, Rotatores

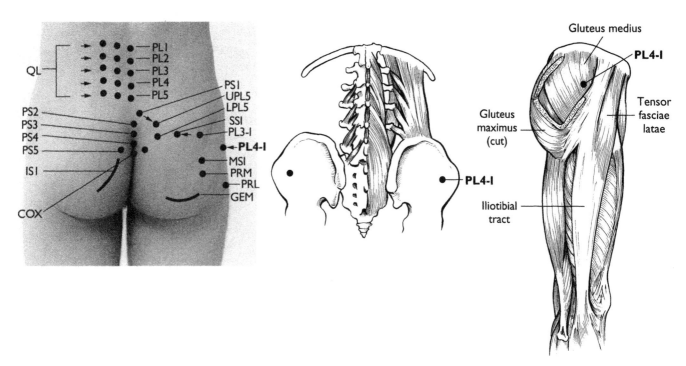

| | | **Location of Tender Point** | This tender point is located approximately 4 cm (1.6 in.) below the crest of the ilium and just posterior to the tensor fascia lata. |

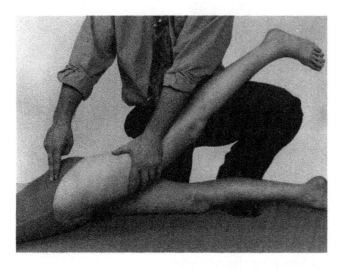 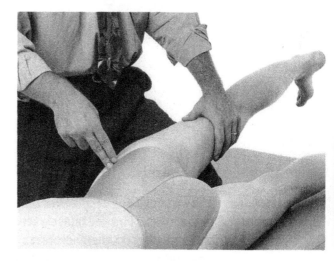

Position of Treatment The patient lies prone while the therapist stands on the same side of the tender point. The therapist then extends the thigh on the affected side and supports it with the therapist's leg or a pillow. The therapist then slightly adducts and moderately externally rotates the thigh.

Note: PL3-I and PL4-I may also be performed in the lateral recumbent position.

LUMBAR SPINE, PELVIS, AND HIP

152. Upper Posterior Fifth Lumbar (UPL5)
Multifidus, Rotatores, SI Ligaments

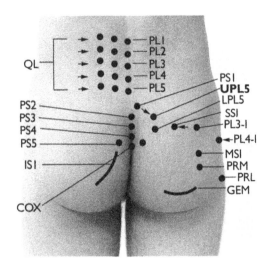
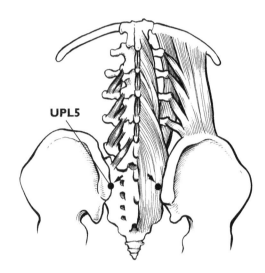

Location of Tender Point	This tender point is located on the superior medial surface of the posterior superior iliac spine. Pressure is applied inferiorly and laterally.

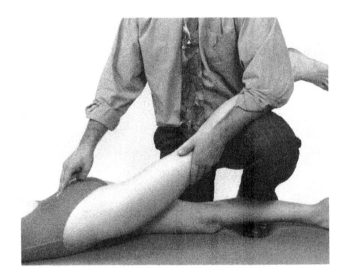
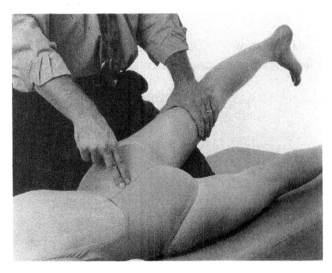

Position of Treatment	The patient lies prone with the therapist standing on the opposite or same side of tenderness. The therapist extends the hip on the affected side and supports the patient's leg on the therapist's thigh. The therapist then slightly adducts the patient's leg and adds mild external rotation to fine-tune the position.

> **Note:** The primary movement is extension. The treatment may also be performed in the lateral recumbent position.

153. Lower Posterior Fifth Lumbar (LPL5)   Iliopsoas, SI Ligaments

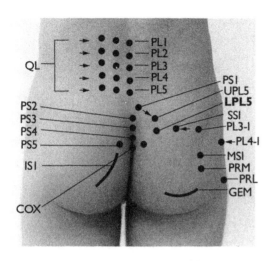

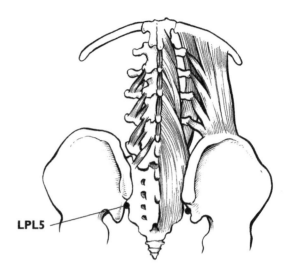

Location of Tender Point   This tender point is located approximately 1.5 cm (0.6 in.) inferior to the posterior superior iliac spine in the sacral notch. Pressure is applied anteriorly.

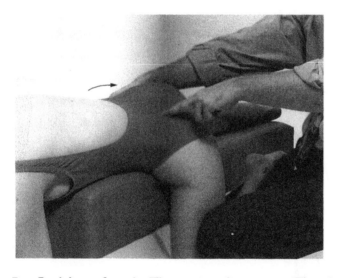

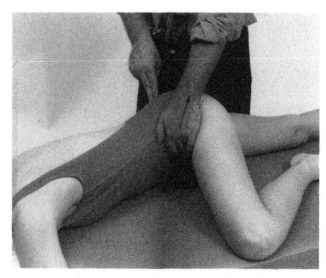

Position of Treatment

1. The patient lies prone. The therapist, seated on the tender point side, asks the patient to move to that side of the table so that the affected leg can be dropped off the edge of the table. The therapist then grasps the ipsilateral leg, flexes the hip to approximately 90°, and adds slight adduction and internal rotation. The opposite ilium may be retracted slightly to fine-tune. Can also be done in side lying with the tender point side up.

2. The patient lies prone. The therapist stands on the opposite side of the tender point and grasps the ilium, at the level of the ASIS, on the side of the tender point. The patient is instructed to flex and abduct the leg on the affected side. The ilium is then retracted and rotated toward the tender point side.

Note: This is a flexion dysfunction with a tender point located posteriorly.

LUMBAR SPINE, PELVIS, AND HIP

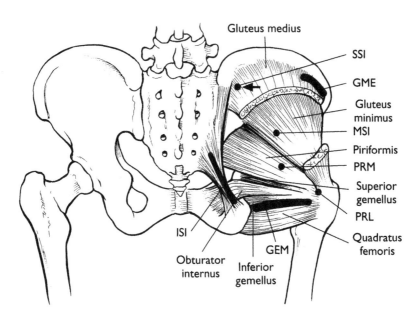

Posterior View

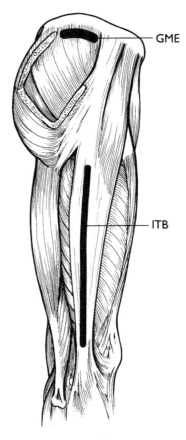

Lateral View

154. Superior Sacroiliac (SSI) Gluteus Medius

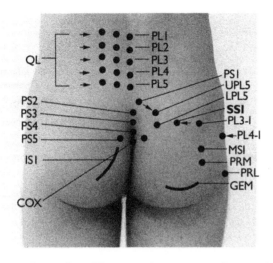 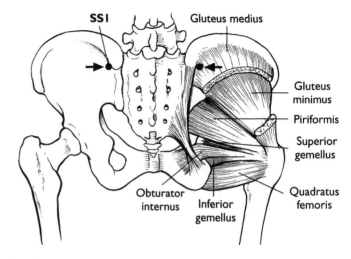

| | **Location of Tender Point** | This tender point is located on the lateral aspect of the posterior superior iliac spine (PSIS). Pressure is applied anteriorly approximately 3 cm (1.2 in.) lateral to the PSIS and then medially. |

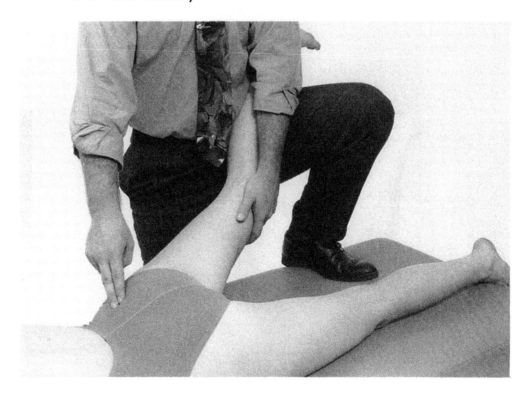

| | **Position of Treatment** | The patient is prone, and the therapist stands on the side of the tender point. The therapist places his or her foot or knee on the table and supports the patient's extended thigh on the therapist's thigh. The hip is moderately extended and slightly abducted. |

155. Middle Sacroiliac (MSI)   Gluteus Minimus

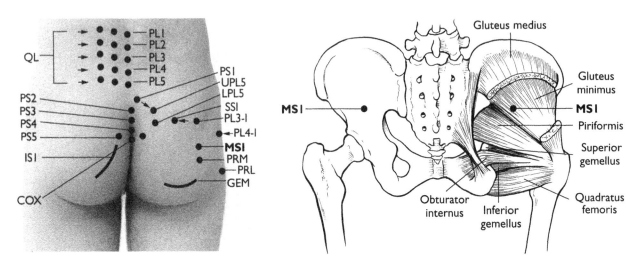

■ **Location of Tender Point**   This tender point is located in the center of the buttocks. Pressure is applied anteriorly and medially.

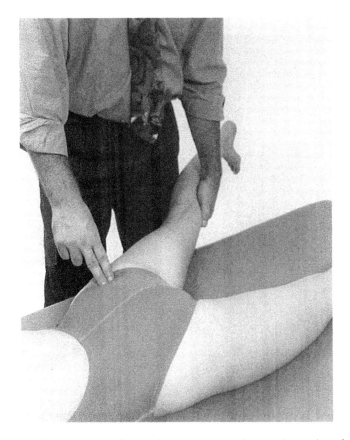

■ **Position of Treatment**   The patient is prone, and the therapist stands on the side of the tender point. The therapist grasps the patient's leg and markedly abducts the thigh. The therapist fine-tunes the position with a slight amount of flexion/extension or internal/external rotation.

156. Inferior Sacroiliac (ISI)   Coccygeus, Sacrotuberous Ligament

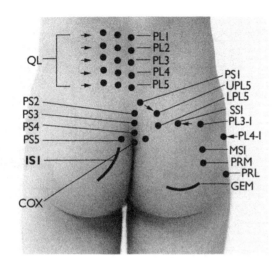
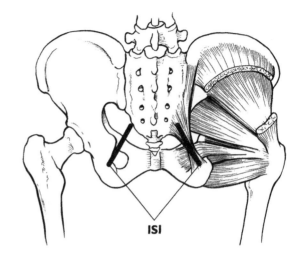

| **Location of Tender Point** | This tender point is located in a line along the sacrotuberous ligament from the ischial tuberosity to the posterior aspect of the inferior lateral angle of the sacrum. Pressure is applied anteriorly and laterally. |

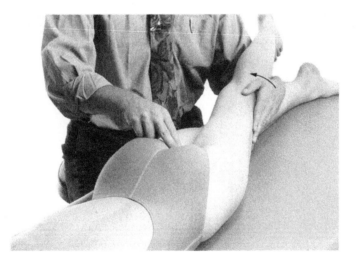

| **Position of Treatment** | The patient is prone with the therapist on the side opposite the tender point. The therapist reaches across to grasp the leg on the involved side and extend, adduct, and externally rotate it across the uninvolved leg. This position may be performed in the lateral recumbent posture with the involved side up. |

157. Gemelli (GEM)   Gemelli, Quadratus Femoris

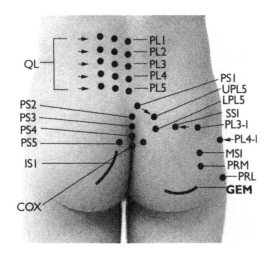
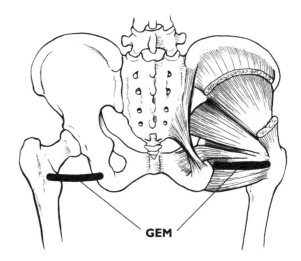

Location of Tender Point   This tender point is located on a line from the lateral inferior surface of the ischial tuberosity to the medial aspect of the posterior surface of the greater trochanter of the femur. This is along the gluteal fold. Pressure is applied anteriorly.

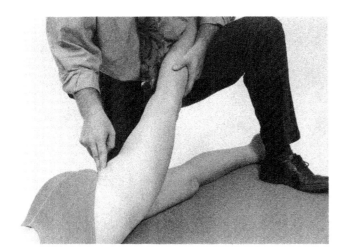
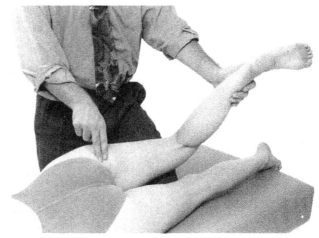

Position of Treatment

1. The patient is prone. The therapist stands on the opposite side of the tender point, places the patient's ankle in the therapist's axilla, and grasps the patient's flexed knee. The therapist extends, adducts, and externally rotates the hip. (See photo above left.)

2. The therapist stands on the same side as the tender point and supports the patient's thigh on the therapist's thigh (which is resting on the table) and produces extension, adduction, and external rotation. (See photo above right.)

158, 159. Piriformis—Medial (PRM)   Piriformis
Piriformis—Lateral (PRL)   Piriformis Insertion

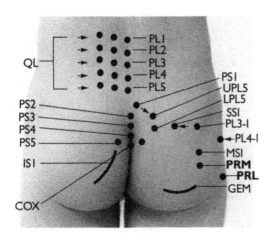 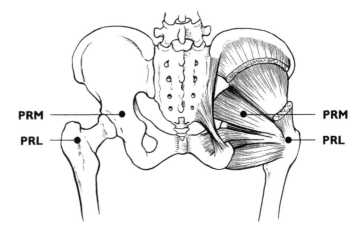

Location of Tender Point (PRM)	This tender point is found in the belly of the piriformis approximately halfway between the inferior lateral angle of the sacrum and the greater trochanter. Pressure is applied anteriorly.
Location of Tender Point (PRL)	This tender point is located on the posterior, superior, lateral surface of the greater trochanter. Pressure is applied anteriorly.

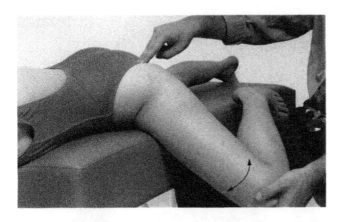 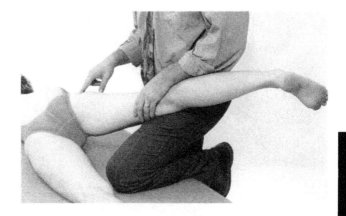

Position of Treatment	1. PRM: The patient is prone, and the therapist is seated on the tender point side. The ipsilateral leg is suspended off the table with the bent knee resting on the therapist's thigh. The hip is flexed to approximately 60° to 90° and abducted. Internal/external rotation is used to fine-tune the position. (See photo above left.)
	2. PRL: The patient is prone, and the therapist stands on the tender point side. The ipsilateral thigh of the patient is extended and abducted and supported on the therapist's thigh, which is resting on the table. The therapist brings the patient's thigh as close as possible to the therapist's hip and then rolls the patient's thigh down toward the table to produce marked external rotation. (See photo above right.) (This treatment may also be used for PRM.)

Note: Piriformis is an external rotator when in extension and an abductor when in flexion.

LUMBAR SPINE, PELVIS, AND HIP

160. Gluteus Medius (GME)

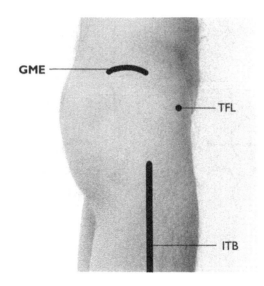

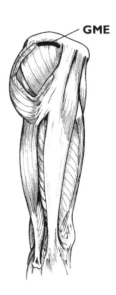

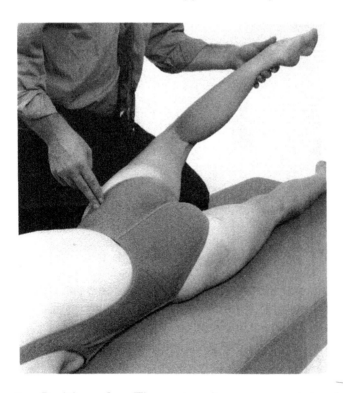

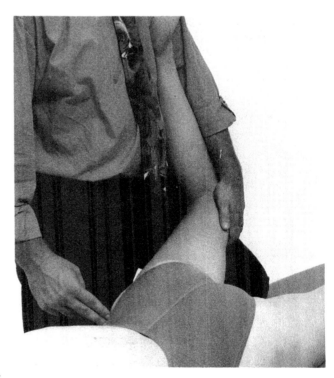

Location of Tender Point These tender points are located on a line approximately 1 cm (0.4 in.) inferior to the iliac crest and 3 to 5 cm (1.2 to 2 in.) on either side of the midaxillary line. Pressure is applied medially.

Position of Treatment The patient lies prone, and the therapist stands on the same side as the tender point. The therapist extends and abducts the hip and supports the patient's leg on the therapist's thigh. The hip is positioned in marked external rotation for tender points located posterior to the midaxillary line (see photo above left) and in internal rotation for those located anterior to the midaxillary line (see photo above right).

161. Iliotibial Band (ITB)

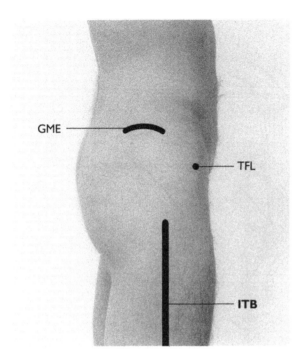

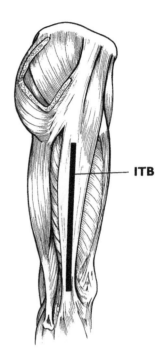

Location of Tender Point	These tender points are located on the iliotibial band along the lateral aspect of the thigh on the midaxillary line. Pressure is applied medially.

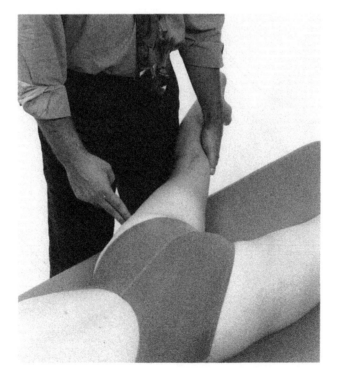

Position of Treatment	The patient may be supine or prone. The therapist stands on the side of the tender point, grasps the patient's leg, and produces marked hip abduction and slight hip flexion with internal or external rotation to fine-tune the position.

POSTERIOR SACRUM *Tender Points*

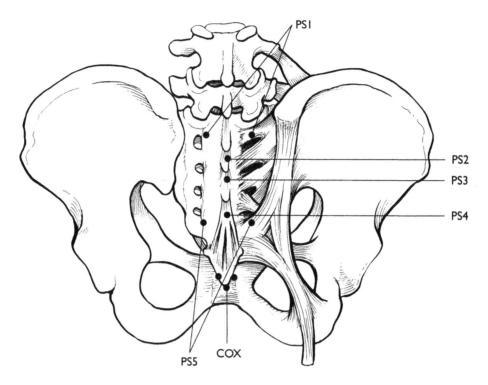

Posterior View

PS1

PS2

PS3

PS4

PS5   COX

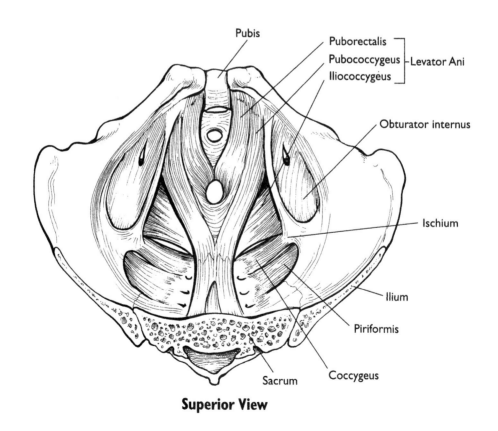

Superior View

Pubis

Puborectalis
Pubococcygeus ⎤ Levator Ani
Iliococcygeus ⎦

Obturator internus

Ischium

Ilium

Piriformis

Sacrum   Coccygeus

162. Posterior First Sacral (PS1)   Levator Ani

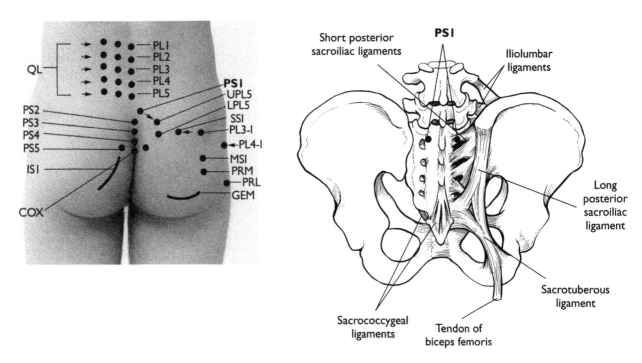

Location of Tender Point   This tender point is located in the sacral sulcus, medial and slightly superior to the PSIS. Pressure is applied anteriorly.

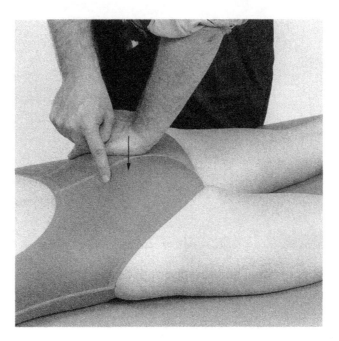

Position of Treatment   The patient is prone. The therapist applies an anterior pressure on the inferior lateral angle opposite the tender point side, resulting in rotation around an oblique axis.

163. Posterior Second Sacral (PS2)   Levator Ani

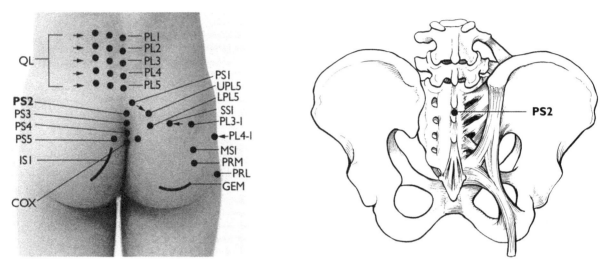

▌ **Location of**   This tender point is located on the midline of the sacrum between the first and
▌ **Tender Point**   second sacral tubercles. Pressure is applied anteriorly.

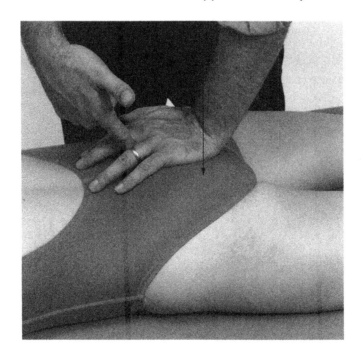

▌ **Position of**   The patient is prone. The therapist applies an anterior pressure on the sacral apex in
▌ **Treatment**   the midline, producing rotation around a transverse axis.

164. Posterior Third Sacral (PS3)   Levator Ani

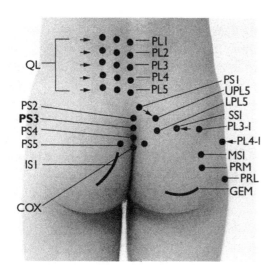
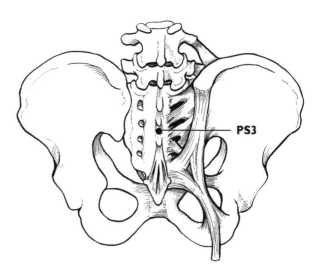

Location of Tender Point	This tender point is located in the midline of the sacrum between the second and third sacral tubercles. Pressure is applied anteriorly.

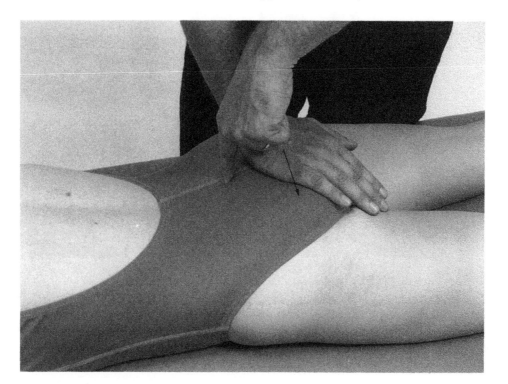

Position of Treatment	The patient is prone. The therapist applies an anterior pressure on the apex (or occasionally the base) of the sacrum in the midline, resulting in rotation around a transverse axis. Alternatively, the patient may be placed in sacral extension by raising the head end of the table and the foot end of the table or by using pillows to support the patient's trunk and lower limbs in extension, with the third sacral segment as the fulcrum.

LUMBAR SPINE, PELVIS, AND HIP

165. Posterior Fourth Sacral (PS4)   Levator Ani

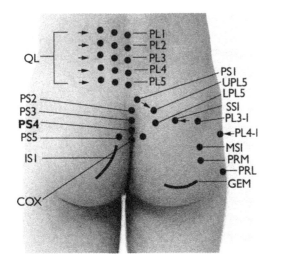
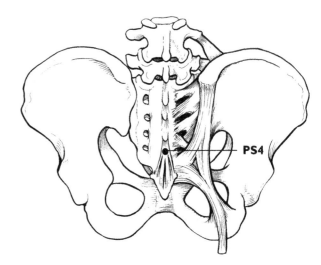

| ¶ **Location of Tender Point** | This tender point is located in the midline of the sacrum just above the sacral hiatus. Pressure is applied anteriorly. |

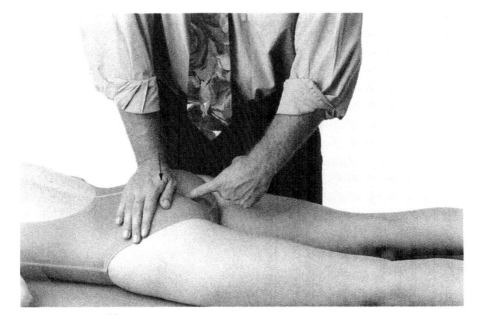

| ¶ **Position of Treatment** | The patient is prone. The therapist applies an anterior pressure on the sacral base in the midline, producing rotation around a transverse axis. |

166. Posterior Fifth Sacral (PS5)   Levator Ani

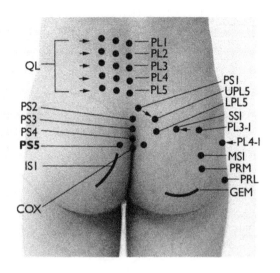

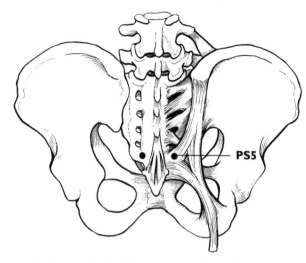

| | Location of Tender Point | This tender point is located approximately 1 cm (0.4 in.) superior and medial to the inferior lateral angle of the sacrum. Pressure is applied anteriorly. |

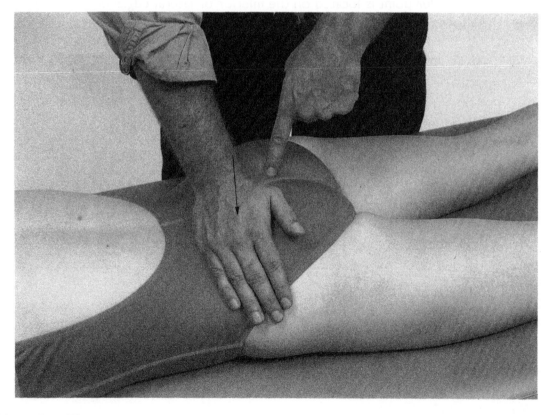

| | Position of Treatment | The patient is prone. The therapist applies an anterior pressure on the sacral base on the side opposite the tender point, resulting in rotation around an oblique axis. |

167. Coccyx (COX)
Pubococcygeus, Sacrotuberous Lig., Sacrospinous Lig.

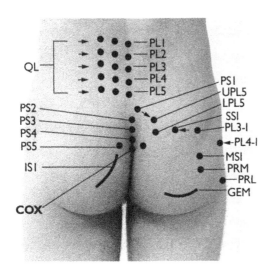 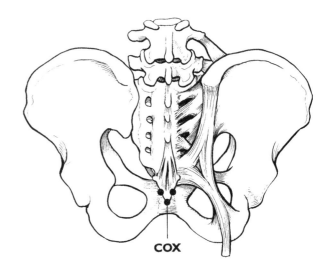

Location of Tender Point This tender point is located on the inferior or lateral edges of the coccyx. Pressure is applied superiorly or medially.

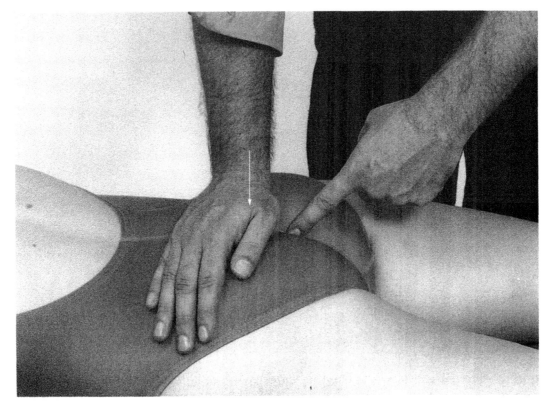

Position of Treatment The patient is prone. The therapist applies an anterior pressure on the sacral apex in the midline. Rotation or lateral flexion of the sacrum, usually toward the tender point side, may be added to fine-tune the position.

LOWER LIMB

⁋Lower Limb Dysfunction

The complex structure and function of the lower limb in weight bearing and gait mechanics is a subject beyond the scope of this text. The bipedal posture has necessitated several adaptations and stability challenges that are not faced by quadrupeds. The knee is often fully extended in standing, and the heel is used as a weight-bearing support, unlike our four-legged counterparts. From a functional point of view, these factors make the lower limb extremely vulnerable to injury. It is important to note that all joint surfaces, including weight-bearing joints such as the knee, are never fully in contact, but are separated by a layer of synovial fluid. The balance of forces around a joint, made up of capsular, ligamentous, and muscular tensions, creates a *tensegrity* structure.[12] The deterioration of joints seen in osteoarthritis and related conditions may be attributable to disruption of the state of balance of the supporting elements and the resultant compression and abrasion of adjacent surfaces.

In addressing lower limb dysfunction, it is recommended that proximal tissues, specifically the lumbar spine and pelvis, be thoroughly examined for significant tender points. When indicated by the severity of these findings, the proximal areas should be treated first. This often obviates the need for direct treatment of the lower limb and thus improves the efficiency of therapy. (See Chapter 4).

Common clinical findings with respect to lower limb dysfunction include general pain, shin splints, jumper's knee, chondromalacia patella, muscle strain (hamstring, gastrocnemius), strain or rupture of the cruciate ligaments or the medial collateral ligament, injury to the medial or lateral meniscus, ankle strain, and foot strain. As mentioned in the section on the lumbar spine and pelvis, deterioration of the arches of the foot is an important factor in low back dysfunction. This may also play an important role in the development of the abnormal biomechanics involved in lower limb conditions.[6]

⁋Treatment

Tender points for the knee and ankle are found around these joints and are often treated by the simple application of folding the joint around the tender point, with varying modifications. The foot can conveniently be divided into three sections: the hindfoot, which has three tender points; the midfoot, which has four tender points; and the forefoot. Palpation of tender points on the plantar surface of the foot requires increased pressure to penetrate the thickened tissue in this region. The knee, ankle, and foot sustain tremendous amounts of force during normal activities, including gait mechanics and simple weight bearing.[20] The structure of these joints reflects this high load demand, and therefore the ligaments and articular soft tissues are extremely thick and resistant to deformation. Thus treatment of the knee, ankle, and foot requires a great deal of force compared with other areas of the body.

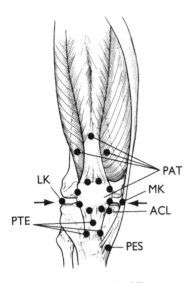

Anterior Muscular View

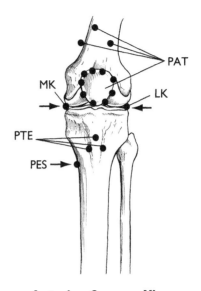

Anterior Osseous View

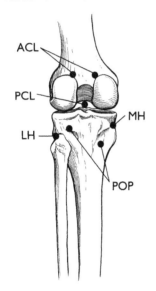

Posterior Osseous View

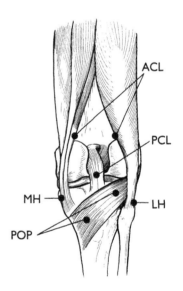

Posterior Muscular View

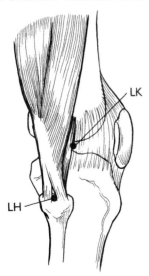

Lateral View

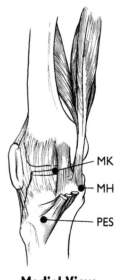

Medial View

168. Patella (PAT)   Quadriceps Femoris, Patellar Retinaculum

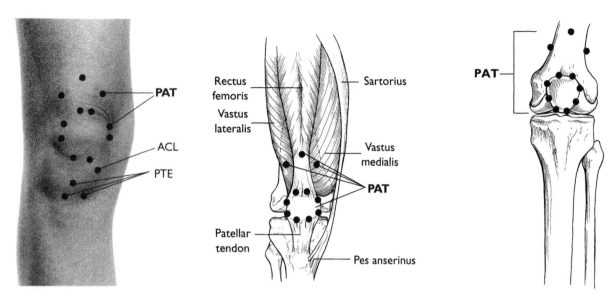

| **Location of Tender Point** | These tender points are located around the periphery of the patella or in the distal belly of the quadriceps femoris. Pressure is applied toward the center of the patella or posteriorly on the quadriceps. Common locations include the superior, lateral, and medial aspects of the patella. |

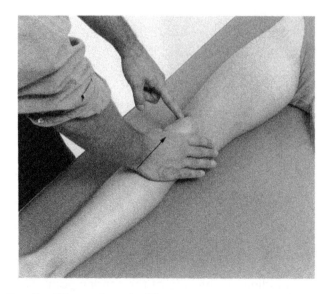 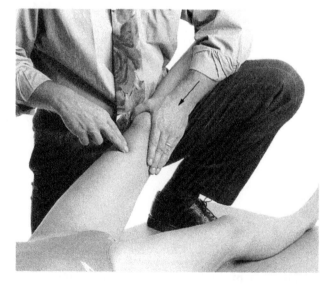

| **Position of Treatment** | 1. The patient is supine. The therapist pushes on the border of the patella on the opposite side of the tender point, pushing the patella toward the tender point. Fine-tuning is accomplished by rotating the patella in a clockwise or counter-clockwise direction. (See photo above left.) |
| | 2. For tender points in the belly of the quadriceps, the involved hip may be flexed to approximately 45° and the knee extended by resting the patient's distal tibia on the therapist's thigh. Fine-tuning is accomplished by rotating the patella in a clockwise or counterclockwise direction. (See photo above right.) |

LOWER LIMB

169. Patellar Tendon (PTE)   Quadriceps Femoris

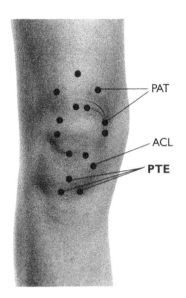
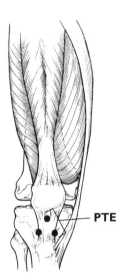
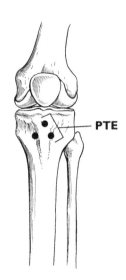

Location of Tender Point
This tender point is located on the sides of the patellar tendon or near the apex of the patella. Pressure is applied by squeezing the tendon between the thumb and fingers.

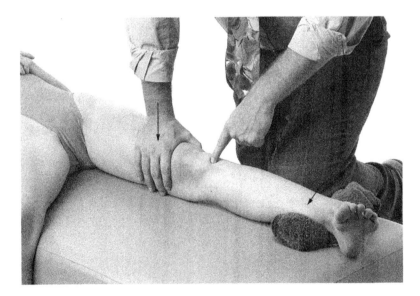

Position of Treatment
The patient is supine with the therapist standing on the side of the tender point. The distal tibia on the involved side is supported on a roll, and the therapist internally rotates the tibia and applies posterior pressure on the distal femur to produce marked hyperextension of the knee.

170. Medial Knee (MK)   Medial Collateral Ligament

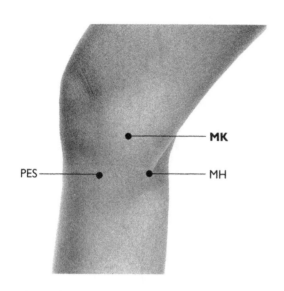

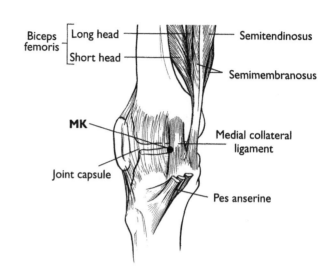

Location of Tender Point   This tender point is located on the medial, midsagittal aspect of the knee along the joint space. Pressure is applied laterally.

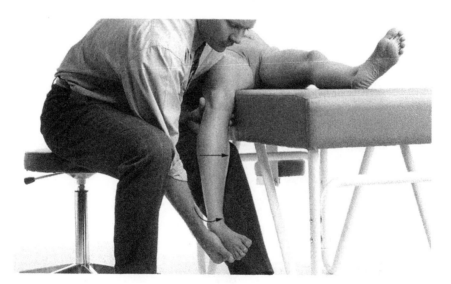

Position of Treatment   The patient lies supine with the affected thigh extended and abducted off the edge of the table. The therapist then flexes the affected knee 40° and adds slight adduction (varus force) and marked internal rotation of the tibia.

Note: Internal rotation of the tibia may be facilitated by stabilizing the patient's femur with the therapist's shoulder and by placing the therapist's tibia against the medial aspect of the patient's calcaneus. The therapist then pushes medially on the lateral aspect of the patient's foot using the therapist's tibia as a fulcrum (as shown above).

LOWER LIMB

171. Lateral Knee (LK)　Lateral Collateral Ligament

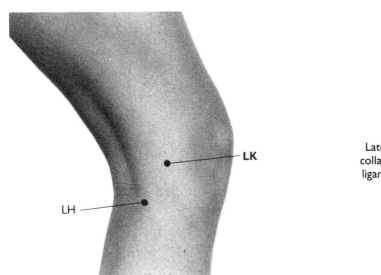

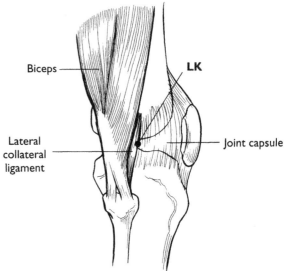

Location of Tender Point　This tender point is located on the lateral, midsagittal aspect of the knee along the joint space. Pressure is applied medially.

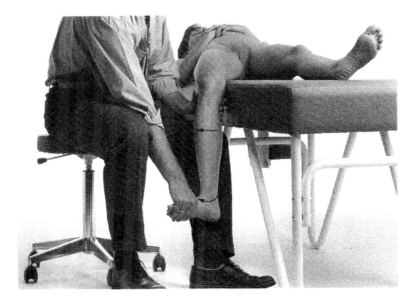

Position of Treatment　The patient lies supine with the affected thigh extended and abducted off the edge of the table. The therapist flexes the affected knee approximately 40° and then either abduct the lower leg (i.e., valgus force to the tibia). The tibia is then externally rotated.

Note: The therapist may use his or her shoulder and tibia for leverage as for MK.

172. Medial Hamstring (MH)

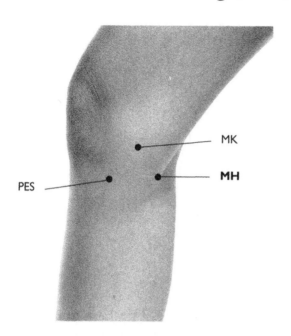
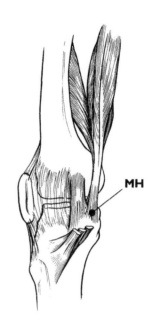

Location of Tender Point This tender point is located on the posterior, medial surface of the tibia, on the tendinous attachments of the semimembranosis and the semitendinosis. Pressure is applied anterolaterally.

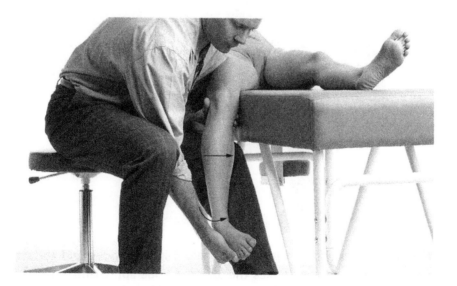

Position of Treatment The patient lies supine with the affected thigh extended and abducted off the edge of the table. The therapist then flexes the affected knee 40° and adds slight adduction (varus force) and marked internal rotation of the tibia.

LOWER LIMB

173. Lateral Hamstring (LH)

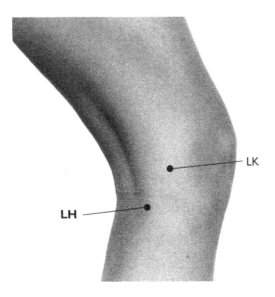
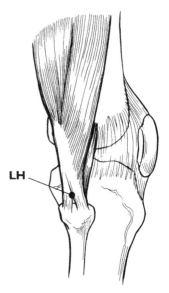

Location of Tender Point This tender point is located on the posterior, lateral surface of the head of the fibula, on the tendinous attachments of the biceps femoris. Pressure is applied anteromedially.

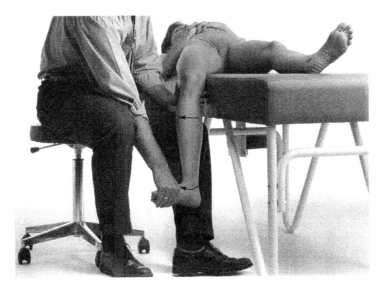

Position of Treatment The patient lies supine with the affected thigh extended and abducted off the edge of the table. The therapist flexes the affected knee approximately 40° and then abduct the lower leg (i.e., valgus force to the tibia). The tibia is then externally rotated.

174. Pes Anserinus (PES)   Pes Anserine Insertion

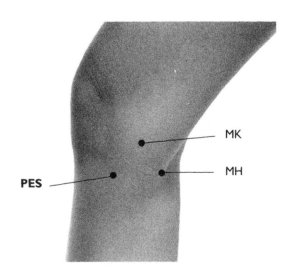
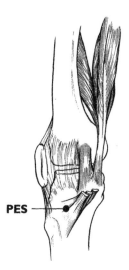

Location of Tender Point   This tender point is located on the anterior, medial aspect of the tibia at the level of and medial to the tibial tuberosity. Pressure is applied posteriorly and laterally.

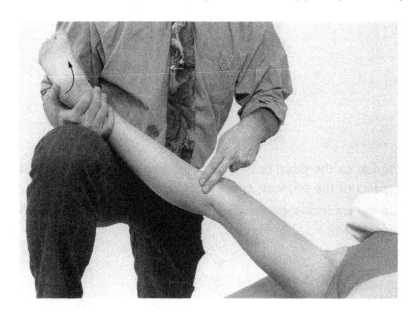

Position of Treatment   The patient is supine with the therapist standing on the side of the tender point. The therapist places his or her foot or knee on the table and supports the patient's tibia. The therapist then flexes the hip 45°, abducts the hip slightly, extends the knee, and externally rotates the tibia.

Note: The treatment for PES does not specifically reproduce the action of the pes anserine muscle group. The designation of the tender point is used only as a landmark. The pes anserine inserts here.

Note: The Medical Hamstring (MH) treatment can also be used.

LOWER LIMB

175. Anterior Cruciate Ligament (ACL)

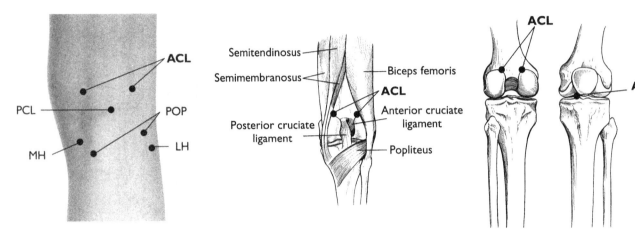

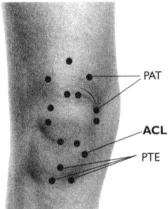

Location of **Tender Point**	1. Median to the distal hamstrings, in the superior-lateral and superior-medial aspects of the popliteal space. Pressure is applied anteriorly.
	2. On the anterior-superior aspect of the proximal tibia. Pressure is applied posteriorly (not shown).

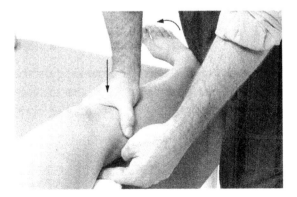

Position of **Treatment**	The patient lies supine with a roll placed under the distal end of the femur. The therapist internally rotates the tibia and then applies a marked posterior force on the proximal end of the tibia (approximately 50 pounds). A folded towel or pad may be used over the tibia for comfort.

176. Posterior Cruciate Ligament (PCL)

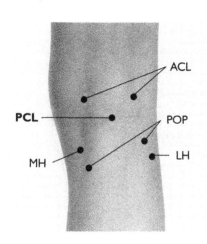

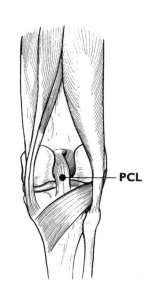

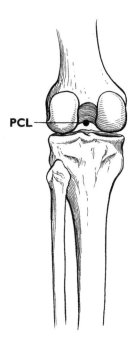

Location of Tender Point   This tender point is located in the center of the popliteal space. Pressure is applied anteriorly.

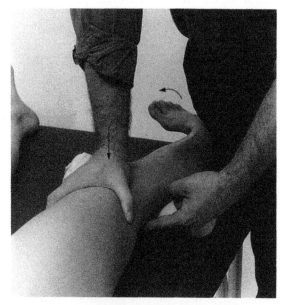

Position of Treatment   The patient lies supine with a roll placed under the proximal end of the tibia on the side of tender point. The therapist internally rotates the tibia and then applies a marked posterior force at the distal end of the femur (approximately 50 pounds).

Note: A folded towel or pad may be used over the femur for comfort. The patient may have pain aggravated by kneeling.

LOWER LIMB

177. Popliteus (POP)

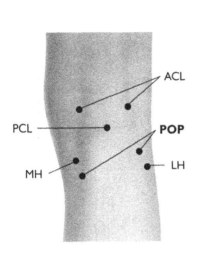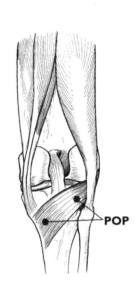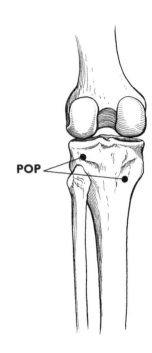

<table>
</table>

Location of Tender Point	1. On the posterior, medial surface of the proximal tibia.
	2. On the lateral aspect of the posterior joint space of the knee. Pressure is applied anteriorly.

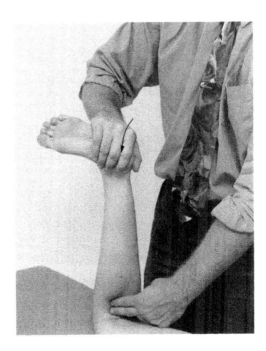

Position of Treatment	The patient is prone. The knee is flexed to 90°, and the therapist grasps the plantar surface of the foot and produces marked internal rotation of the tibia while adding a moderate amount of compression through the knee joint.

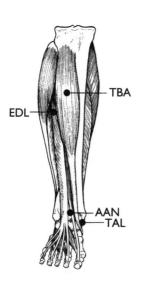

Anterior Muscular View

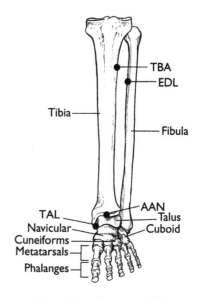

Anterior Osseous View

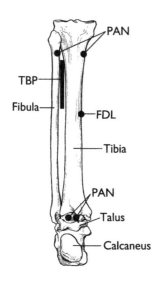

Posterior Osseous View

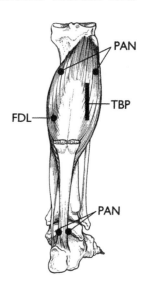

Posterior Muscular View

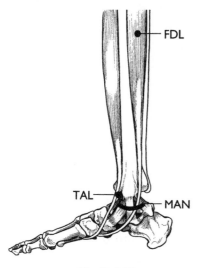

Medial View

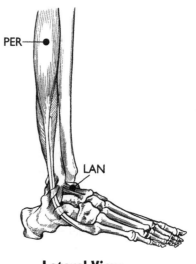

Lateral View

178. Medial Ankle (MAN) Deltoid Ligament

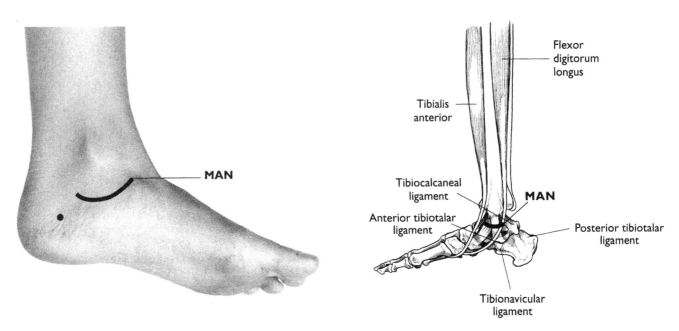

Flexor
digitorum
longus

Tibialis
anterior

Tibiocalcaneal
ligament

Anterior tibiotalar
ligament

MAN

Posterior tibiotalar
ligament

Tibionavicular
ligament

MAN

Location of Tender Point The tender point for the deltoid ligament is located approximately 2 cm (0.8 in.) inferior to the medial malleolus in an arc approximately 2 cm long. Palpate the anterior, middle, and posterior fibers in "horse shoe" fashion. Pressure is applied laterally.

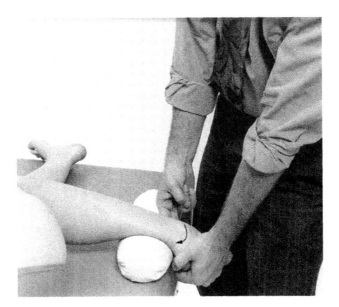

Position of Treatment The patient lies on the uninvolved side with the affected knee flexed and the involved ankle suspended over the edge of the table. A roll or towel is placed under the distal end of the tibia. The upside ankle is treated. The therapist stands behind the patient near the foot end of the table, grasps the calcaneus, and applies a marked floorward force to invert the ankle and fold the foot over the tender point. The proximal end of the involved tibia may need to be supported to limit external rotation at the hip. Internal rotation of the ankle may be added as a fine-tuning measure.

179. Lateral Ankle (LAN)   Anterior Talofibular Ligament

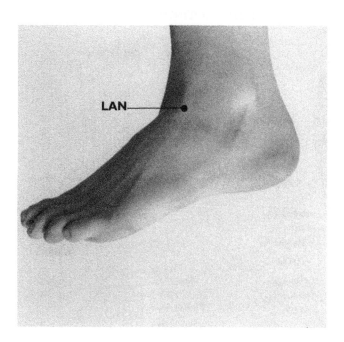 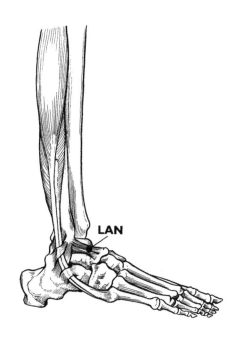

Location of Tender Point   The tender point for the anterior talofibular ligament is located approximately 2 cm (0.8 in.) anterior and inferior to the lateral malleolus in a depression on the talus. Pressure is applied medially.

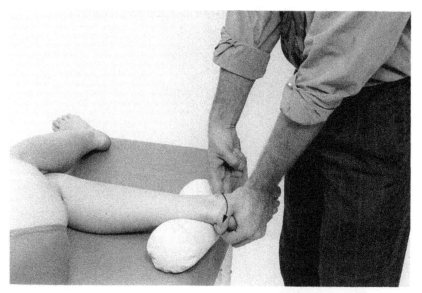

Position of Treatment   The patient lies on the involved side with knees flexed and the involved ankle suspended over the edge of the table. A roll or towel is placed under the distal end of the fibula. The downside ankle is treated. The therapist stands behind the patient near the foot of the table, grasps the calcaneus, and applies a marked floorward force to evert the ankle, thus folding the foot over the tender point. External rotation of the ankle may be added as a fine-tuning measure.

180. Anterior Ankle (AAN)
Extensor Hallucis Longus, Extensor Digitorum Longus

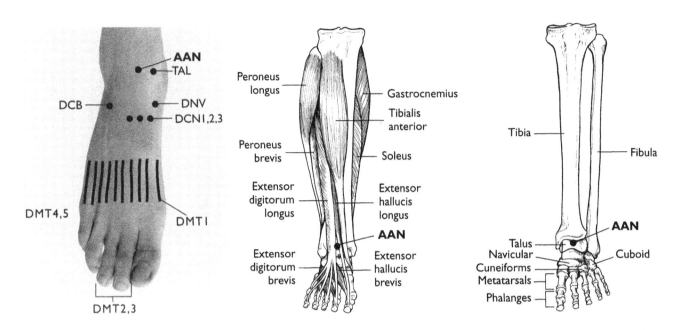

Location of Tender Point	This tender point is located on the anterior aspect of the ankle (talus) between the tendon of the tibialis anterior and the extensor digitorum longus. Dorsiflexion of the ankle may be required to find this point. Once the location is found, release the dorsiflexion to evaluate the TP. Pressure is applied posteriorly.

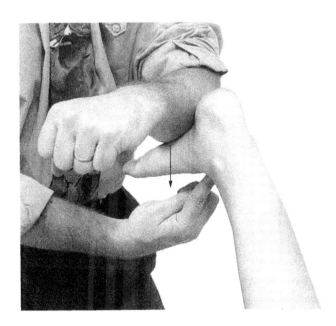

Position of Treatment	The patient is prone with the knee flexed. The therapist stands at the foot end of the table and places his or her forearm across the plantar surface of the midfoot and applies a significant force to produce marked dorsiflexion.

181. Talus (TAL)   Tibialis Anterior

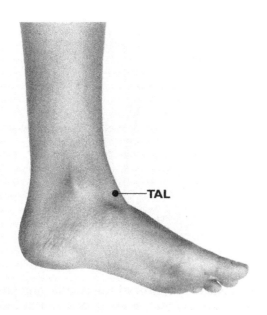

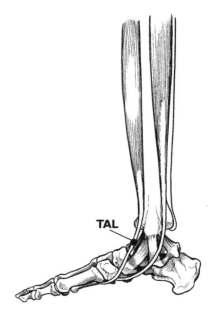

Location of Tender Point   This tender point is located medial to the tibialis anterior tendon in a depression on the talus, approximately 2 cm (0.8 in.) anterior and caudal to the medial malleolus. Pressure is applied laterally.

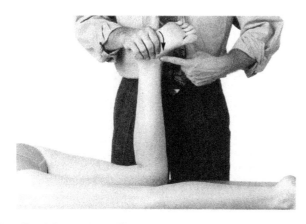

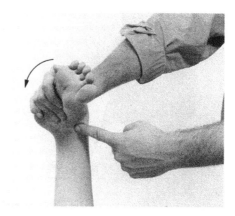

Position of Treatment   The patient is prone with the knee flexed. The therapist stands on the involved side, grasps the foot, and produces marked inversion and internal rotation.

182. Posterior Ankle (PAN)   Gastrocnemius, Soleus

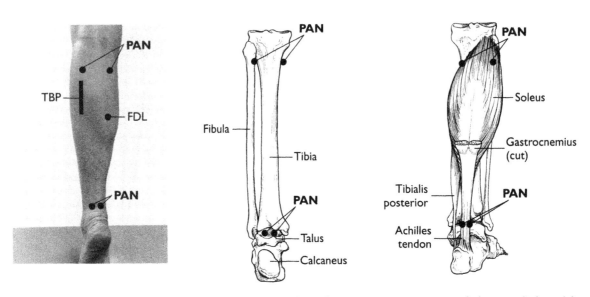

Location of Tender Point   These tender points are located in the superior portion of the medial and lateral heads of the gastrocnemius muscle approximately 2 to 3 cm (0.8 to 1.2 in.) below the knee (pressure applied anteriorly). Another location for tender points is along the sides of the Achilles tendon (pressure applied by squeezing between thumb and fingers).

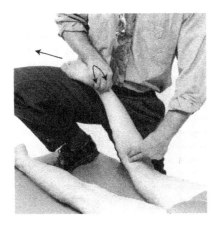
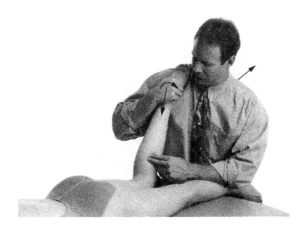

Position of Treatment   The patient is prone. The therapist stands on the side of the tender point, places his or her foot or knee on the table, and supports the dorsum of the patient's foot on the therapist's upper thigh. The therapist produces marked plantar flexion by compressing the calcaneus cephalad toward the tender point and caudal traction by shifting the supporting thigh away from the tender point. Internal rotation of the tibia is used to fine-tune the position.

Note: An alternative treatment may be performed by placing the dorsum of the foot on the therapist's shoulder and grasping the calcaneus with both hands, pressing floorward, fine-tuning with internal rotation.

183. Tibialis Posterior (TBP)

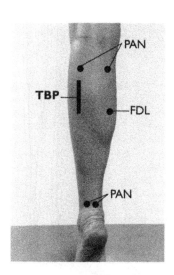

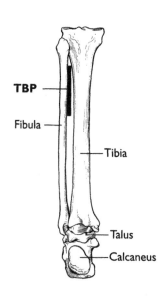

Location of Tender Point	This tender point is located on a median line on the posterior aspect of the calf, between the tibia and fibula from 2 cm (0.8 in.) inferior to the head of the fibula and extending down to the midpoint of the leg. Pressure is applied anteriorly by sinking the fingers gently between the bellies of the gastrocnemius.

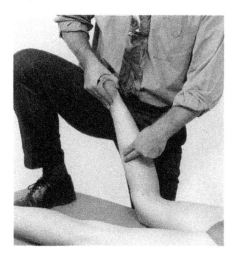

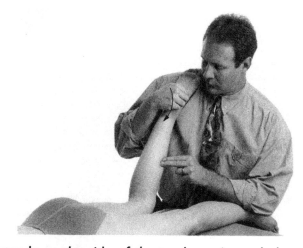

Position of Treatment	The patient is prone. The therapist stands on the side of the tender point and places his or her foot or knee on the table. The dorsum of the patient's foot is placed on the therapist's thigh, the ankle is placed in marked plantar flexion, and the navicular is inverted with respect to the distal foot. Alternatively, the therapist's shoulder may be used to support the dorsum of the foot.

Note: Photo shows practitioner monitoring tender point for FDL. Monitor tender point as described above.

LOWER LIMB

184. Flexor Digitorum Longus (FDL)

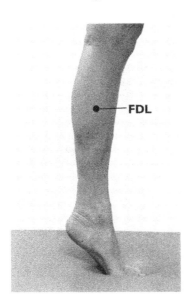 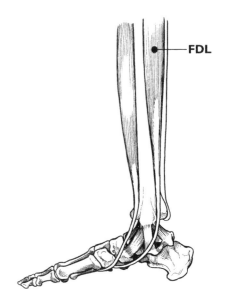

Location of Tender Point This tender point is located posterior to the medial aspect of the tibia near the midpoint of the leg, in the belly of the flexor digitorum longus. Pressure is applied anteriorly and laterally.

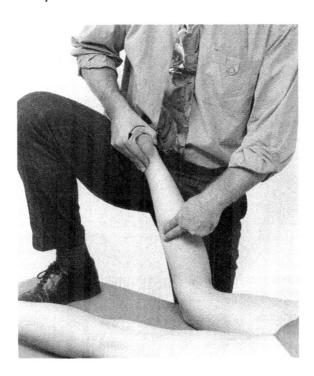

Position of Treatment The patient is prone. The therapist stands on the side of the tender point and places his or her foot or knee on the table. The dorsum of the patient's foot is placed on the therapist's thigh, the ankle is placed in marked plantar flexion, and the calcaneus is inverted with respect to the distal foot. Alternatively, the therapist's shoulder may be used to support the dorsum of the foot.

185. Tibialis Anterior (TBA)

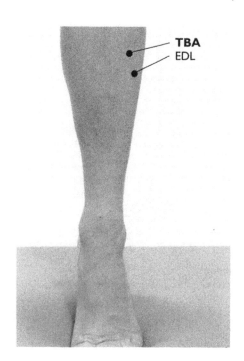

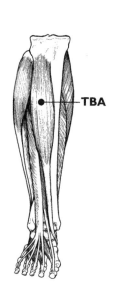

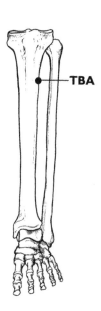

Location of Tender Point
This tender point is located on the tibialis anterior, midway up the leg approximately 2 cm (0.8 in.) lateral to the anterior edge of the tibia. Pressure is applied posteriorly.

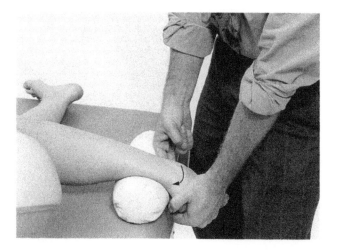

Position of Treatment
The patient lies on the uninvolved side with the affected knee flexed and the involved ankle suspended over the edge of the table. A roll or towel is placed under the distal end of the tibia. The upside ankle is treated. The therapist stands behind the patient near the foot end of the table, grasps the calcaneus, and applies a marked floorward force to invert the ankle and fold the foot over the tender point. The proximal end of the involved tibia may need to be supported to limit external rotation at the hip. Internal rotation of the ankle may be added as a fine-tuning measure.

Note: Photo shows practitioner monitoring tender points for MAN. Monitor tender points as described above.

LOWER LIMB

186. Peroneus (PER)   Peroneus Longus, Brevis

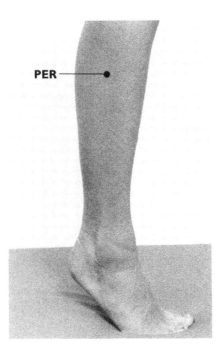

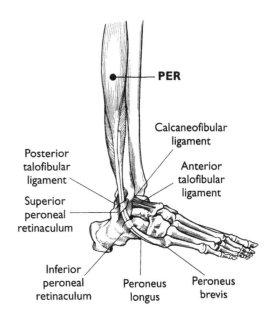

| **Location of Tender Point** | This tender point is located in the belly of the peroneus or on the proximal head of the fibula. Pressure is applied medially. |

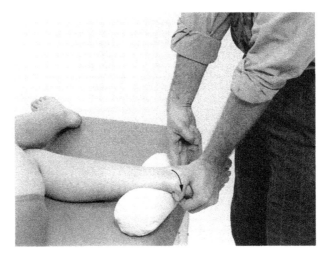

| **Position of Treatment** | The patient lies on the involved side with knees flexed and the involved ankle suspended over the edge of the table. A roll or towel is placed under the distal end of the fibula. The downside ankle is treated. The therapist stands behind the patient near the foot of the table, grasps the calcaneus, and applies a marked forward force to evert the ankle, thus folding the foot over the tender point. External rotation of the ankle may be added as a fine-tuning measure. |

Note: Photo shows practitioner monitoring tender point for LAN. Monitor tender point as described above.

187. Extensor Digitorum Longus (EDL)

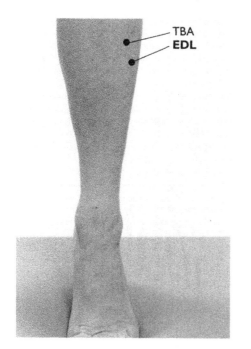

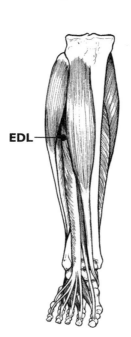

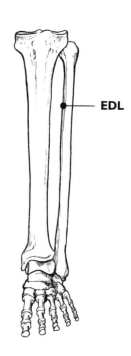

Location of Tender Point   This tender point is located in the belly of the muscle, just lateral to the tibialis anterior, extending from approximately 4 cm (1.6 in.) below the head of the fibula to just above the ankle joint. Pressure is applied posteriorly.

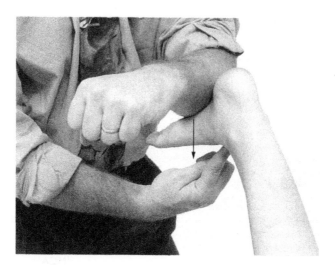

Position of Treatment   The patient is prone with the knee flexed. The therapist stands at the foot end of the table and places his or her forearm across the plantar surface of the midfoot and applies a significant force to produce marked dorsiflexion.

Note: Photo shows practitioner monitoring tender point for AAN. Monitor tender point as described above.

LOWER LIMB

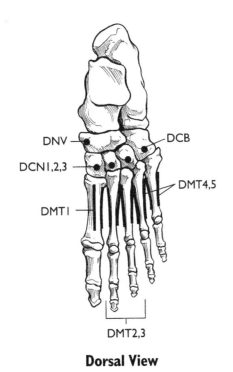

DNV
DCN1,2,3
DMT1
DCB
DMT4,5
DMT2,3

Dorsal View

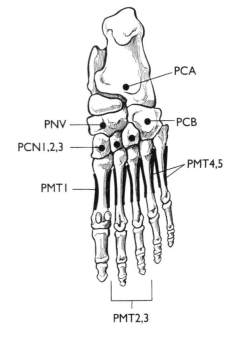

PCA
PNV
PCN1,2,3
PMT1
PCB
PMT4,5
PMT2,3

Plantar View

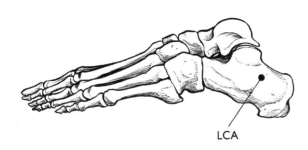

LCA

Lateral View

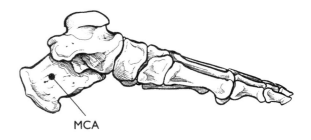

MCA

Medial View

188. Medial Calcaneus (MCA)   Talocalcaneal Joint

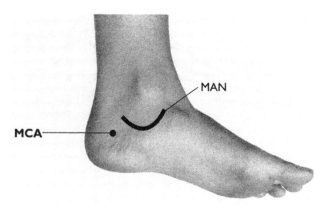

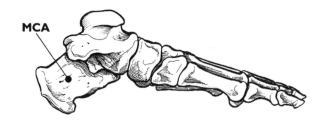

Location of Tender Point   This tender point is located on the medial aspect of the hindfoot approximately 3 cm (1.2 in.) caudal and posterior to the medial malleolus. Pressure is applied laterally.

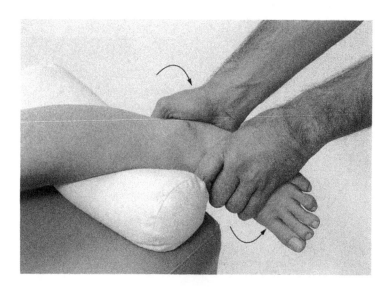

Position of Treatment   The patient lies on the uninvolved side with the affected knee flexed and the involved ankle suspended over the edge of the table. A roll or towel is placed under the distal end of the tibia. The therapist stands behind the patient, contacts the lateral aspect of the affected calcaneus, and applies a marked force to invert the ankle. With the other hand the therapist grasps the midfoot of the patient, as close as possible to the other hand, and forces the midfoot into marked eversion.

189. Lateral Calcaneus (LCA)   Talocalcaneal Joint

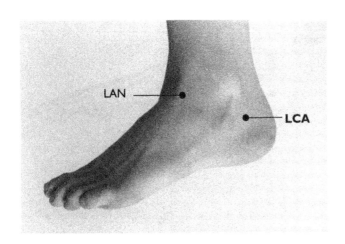

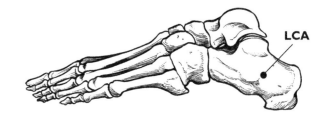

Location of Tender Point	This tender point is located on the lateral aspect of the hindfoot approximately 3 cm (1.2 in.) caudal and posterior to the lateral malleolus. Pressure is applied medially.

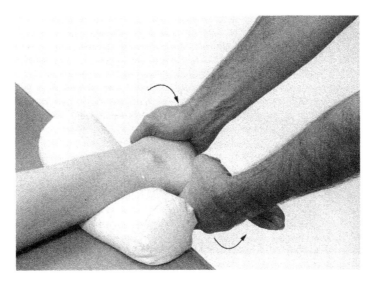

Position of Treatment	The patient lies on the involved side with the affected knee flexed and the involved ankle suspended over the edge of the table. A roll or towel is placed under the distal end of the fibula. The therapist stands behind the patient, contacts the medial aspect of the calcaneus, and applies a marked force to evert the ankle. With the other hand the therapist grasps the midfoot of the patient, as close as possible to the other hand, and forces the midfoot into marked inversion.

190. Plantar Calcaneus (PCA)   Quadratus Plantae, Flexor Digitorum Brevis, Plantar Fascia

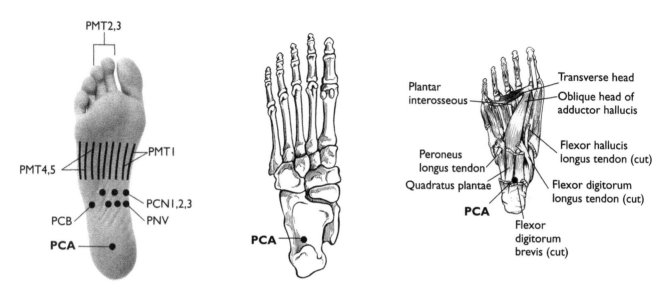

Location of Tender Point	This tender point is located on the plantar surface of the foot, at the anterior end of the calcaneus and along the plantar fascia. Pressure is applied in a cephalad direction.

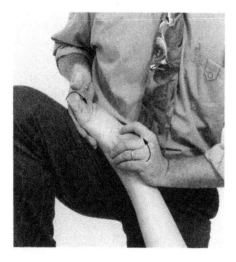 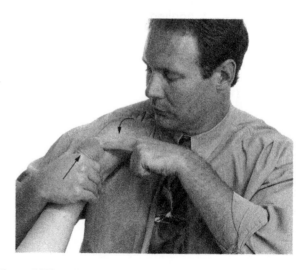

Position of Treatment	The patient is prone with the knee flexed. The therapist stands on the side of the tender point with his or her foot on the table. The dorsum of the patient's foot rests on the therapist's thigh with the distal metatarsals supported into plantar flexion by the therapist's hand. The therapist grasps the dorsum of the calcaneus with the other hand and forces it into dorsiflexion, thus folding the foot over the tender point. Varus or valgus force is used to fine-tune the position. (See photo above left.) An alternative treatment may be performed by supporting the dorsum of the foot on the therapist's shoulder and lifting the calcaneus into plantar flexion. (See photo above right.)

LOWER LIMB

191. Dorsal Cuboid (DCB)   Dorsal Calcaneocuboid Ligament

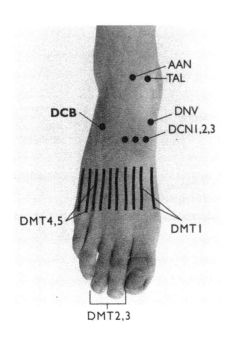

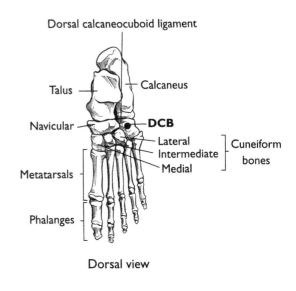

Dorsal view

| **Location of Tender Point** | This tender point is located on the dorsum of the foot, medial and proximal to the proximal head of the fifth metatarsal on the dorsal surface of the cuboid. Pressure is applied caudally. |

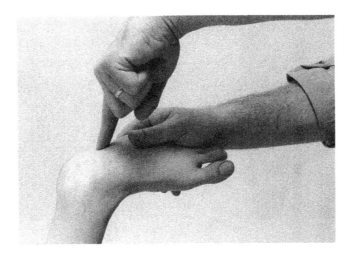

| **Position of Treatment** | The patient is prone with the involved knee flexed. The therapist graps the proximal ends of the fourth and fifth metatarsals and the cuboid and applies an inversion force to the lateral aspect of the foot. This position folds the foot *away* from the tender point. |

192. Plantar Cuboid (PCB)   Plantar Calcaneocuboid Ligament

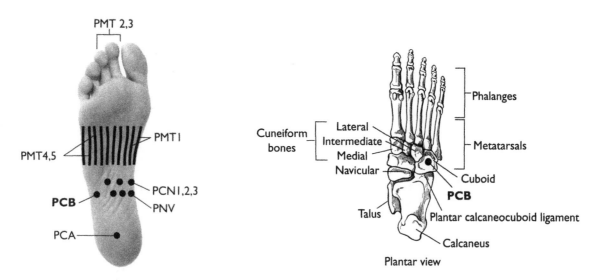

| | Location of Tender Point | This tender point is located on the plantar surface of the cuboid, just medial and proximal to the proximal head of the fifth metatarsal. Pressure is applied in a cephalad direction. |

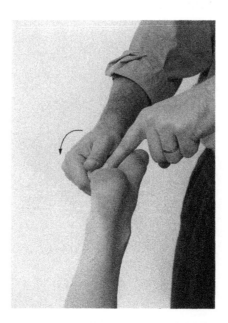

| | Position of Treatment | The patient lies prone with the involved knee flexed. The therapist grasps the proximal ends of the fourth and fifth metatarsals and the cuboid and applies an eversion force to the lateral aspect of the foot. |

193. Dorsal Navicular (DNV)   Talonavicular Ligament

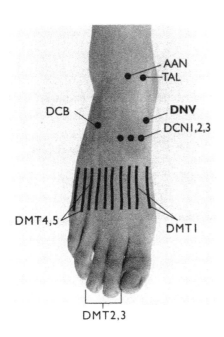

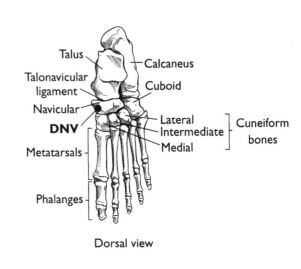

Dorsal view

▌ **Location of Tender Point**   This tender point is located on the dorsal surface of the navicular, near the apex of the medial arch of the foot. Pressure is applied caudally.

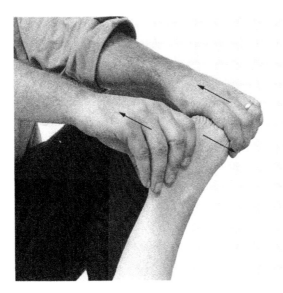

▌ **Position of Treatment**   The patient is prone with the involved knee flexed. The therapist stands on the side of the tender point and places his or her knee against the lateral aspect of the calcaneal-cuboid joint. A towel or pad may be used for comfort. The therapist grasps the medial aspect of the first metatarsal and the medial aspect of the calcaneus and, using the knee as a fulcrum, pulls the forefoot and hindfoot into valgus. This force folds the foot *away* from the tender point.

194. Plantar Navicular (PNV)   Plantar Calcaneonavicular Ligament

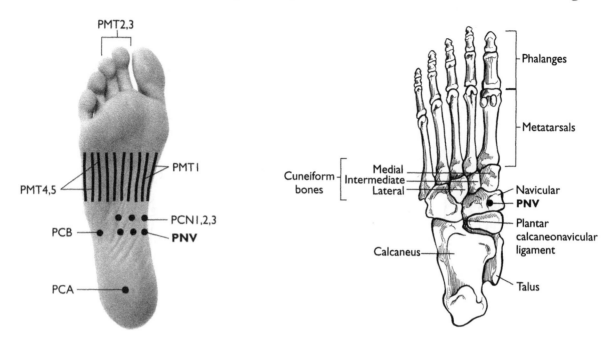

| **Location of Tender Point** | This tender point is located on the plantar surface of the navicular, near the apex of the medial arch of the foot. Pressure is applied in a cephalad direction. |

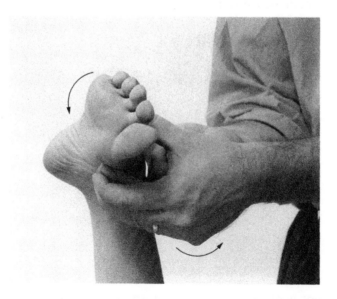

| **Position of Treatment** | The patient is prone with the involved knee flexed. The therapist stands on the side of the tender point and grasps the medial arch of the foot with both hands, reaching over the dorsum of the foot and anterior to the tibia. The therapist's elbows are held close together in front of the therapist's abdomen. The second finger of the distal hand is placed over the plantar surface of the navicular bone, and this contact is reinforced with the first or third finger of the same hand and one or more fingers of the other hand. Force is applied by pulling toward the therapist to produce marked inversion of the foot and plantar flexion of the forefoot. |

LOWER LIMB

195-197. Dorsal First, Second, and Third Cuneiform (DCN1, 2, 3) Dorsal Cuneonavicular Ligament

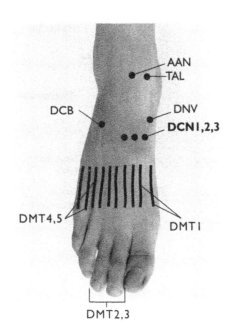

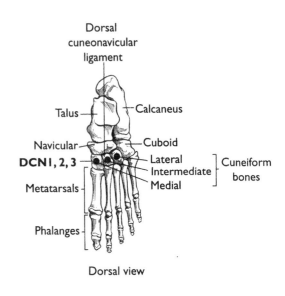

Dorsal view

Location of Tender Point   These tender points are located on the dorsal surface of the first, second, or third cuneiform. Pressure is applied in a caudal direction.

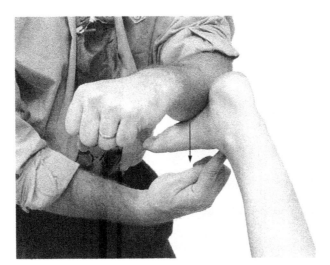

Position of Treatment   The patient is prone with the involved knee flexed. The therapist grasps the first, second or third metatarsal and applies a downward pressure to produce marked dorsiflexion to the level of the cuneiform. Fine-tuning is accomplished with the addition of rotation or side bending of the metatarsals.

198-200. Plantar First, Second, and Third Cuneiform (PCN1, 2, 3)   Plantar Cuneonavicular Ligament

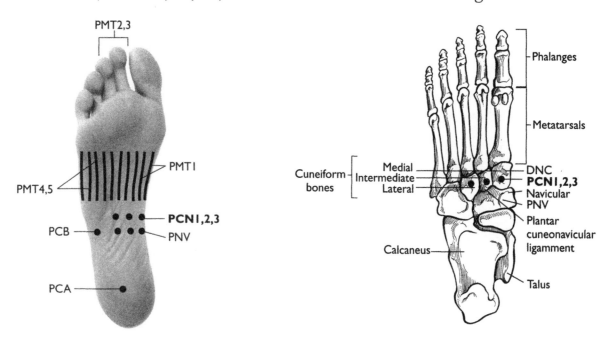

Location of Tender Point	These tender points are located on the plantar surface of the first, second, or third cuneiform. Pressure is applied in a cephalad direction.

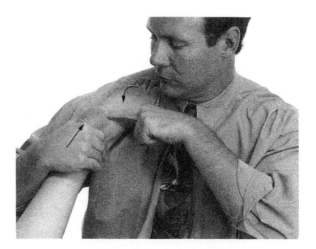

Position of Treatment	The patient is prone with the involved knee flexed and the dorsum of the foot resting on the therapist's thigh or shoulder. The therapist produces marked plantar flexion to the level of the involved cuneiform. Fine-tuning is accomplished with the addition of rotation or side bending of the metatarsals and dorsiflexion of the calcaneus.

201. Dorsal First Metatarsal (DMT1)   Extensor Hallucis Longus

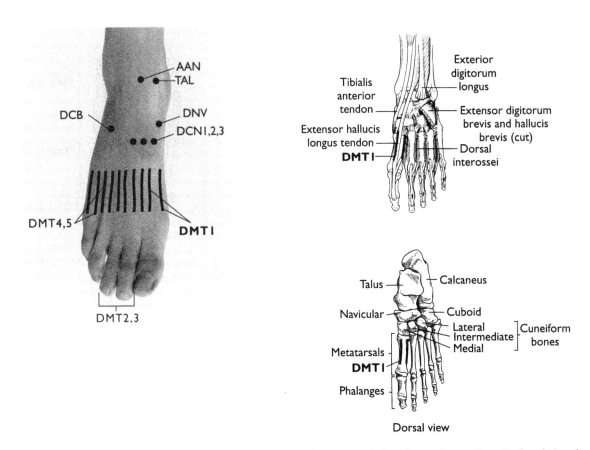

Dorsal view

Location of Tender Point   This tender point is located on the dorsum of the foot along the shaft of the first metatarsal. Pressure is applied caudally and medially.

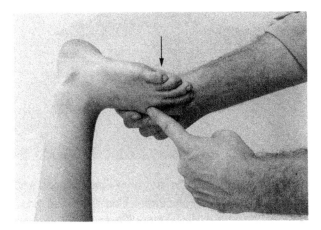

Position of Treatment   The patient is prone with the involved knee flexed. The therapist grasps the distal end of the first metatarsal and applies a downward pressure to produce marked dorsiflexion. Eversion and rotation are added for fine-tuning.

202, 203. Dorsal Second and Third Metatarsals (DMT2, 3)
Extensor Digitorum Longus/Brevis, Dorsal Interossei

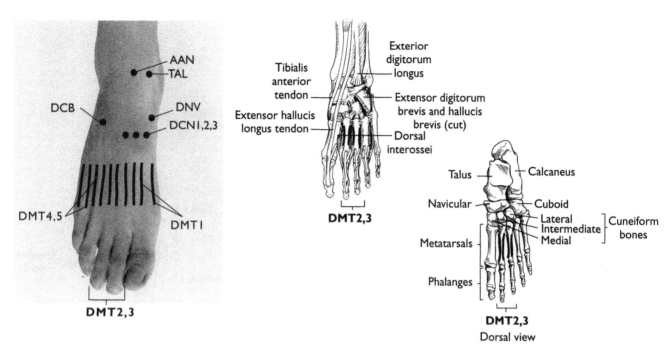

Location of Tender Point These tender points are located on the dorsum of the foot, along the medial or lateral aspects of the shafts of the second and third metatarsals. Pressure is applied caudally and medially or laterally.

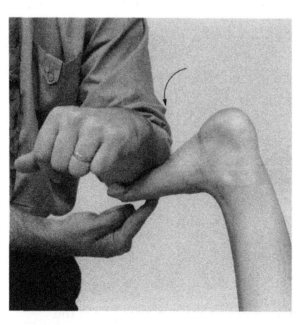
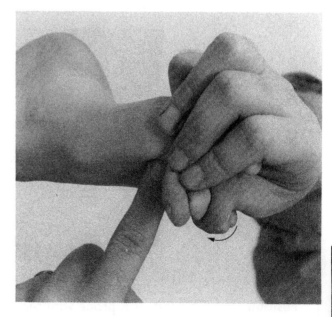

Position of Treatment The patient is prone with the involved knee flexed. The therapist applies a downward pressure on the heads of the second and third metatarsals to produce marked dorsiflexion. Rotation is used to fine-tune the position. (See photo above left.) Occasionally the toes need to be crossed to treat this lesion. (See photo above right.)

204, 205. Dorsal Fourth and Fifth Metatarsals (DMT4, 5)
Extensor Digitorum Longus/Brevis, Dorsal Interossei, Peroneus Tertius

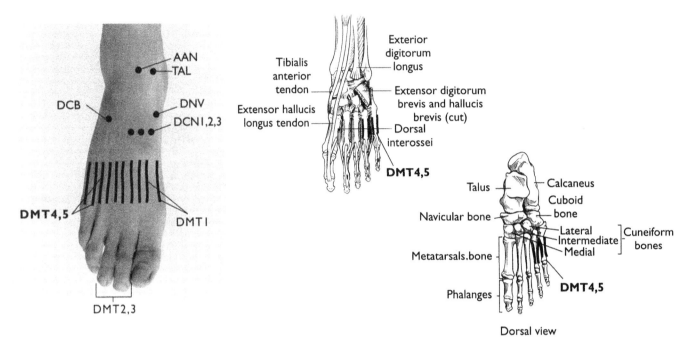

■ **Location of Tender Point**   These tender points are found on the dorsum of the foot along the medial or lateral aspects of the shafts of the fourth metatarsal and along the medial aspect of the shaft of the fifth metatarsal. Pressure is applied caudally and medially or laterally.

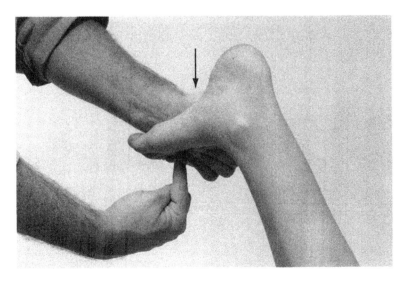

■ **Position of Treatment**   The patient is prone with the involved knee flexed. The therapist grasps the distal ends of the fourth and fifth metatarsals and produces eversion, dorsiflexion, and rotation.

206. Plantar First Metatarsal (PMT1)
Flexor Hallucis Brevis, Adductor Hallucis, Plantar Interossei

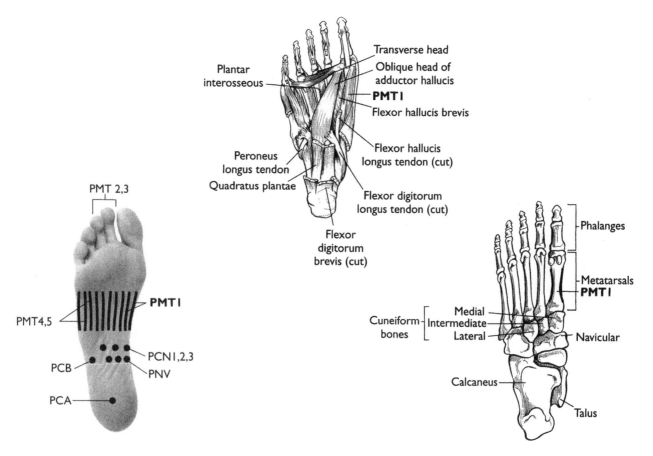

Location of Tender Point	This tender point is located along the lateral side of the plantar surface of the shaft of the first metatarsal. Pressure is applied medially and in a cephalad direction.

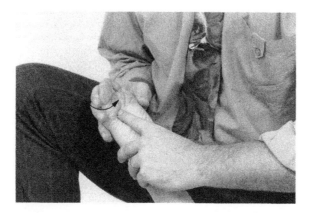

Position of Treatment	The patient is prone with the involved knee flexed and the dorsum of the foot resting on the therapist's knee. The therapist grasps the distal end of the first metatarsal and rolls it into eversion. Internal or external rotation is used to fine-tune the position.

LOWER LIMB

207, 208. Plantar Second and Third Metatarsals (PMT2, 3)
Flexor Digitorum Brevis, Lumbricals, Plantar Interossei

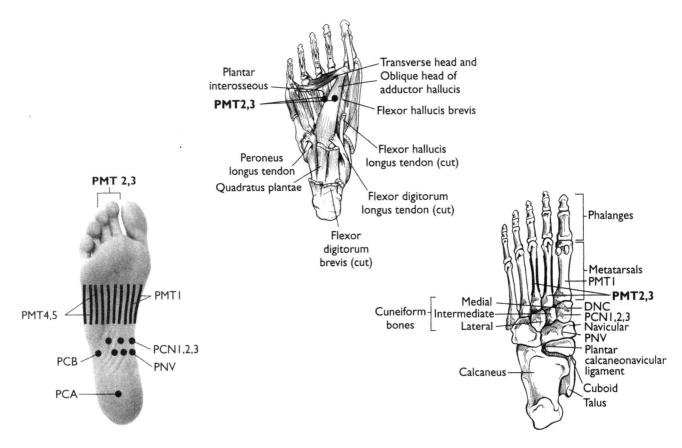

Location of Tender Point

These tender points are located on the plantar surface of the foot along the medial or lateral aspects of the shafts of the second and third metatarsals. Pressure is applied in a cephalad and medial or lateral direction.

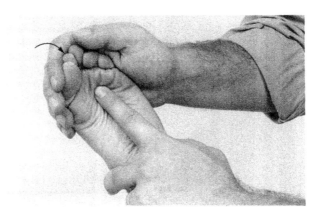

Position of Treatment

The patient is prone with the involved knee flexed and the dorsum of the foot resting on the therapist's thigh. The therapist grasps the distal end of the metatarsals and produces marked plantar flexion. Internal or external rotation is used to fine-tune the position.

209, 210. Plantar Fifth Metatarsal (PMT4, 5)
Flexor Digiti Minimi Brevis, Plantar Interossei

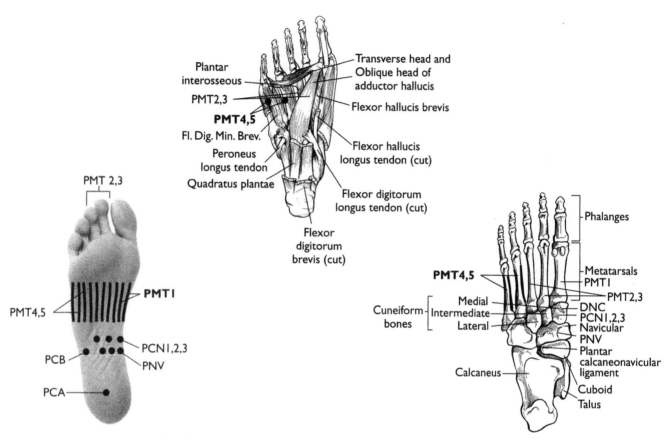

Location of Tender Point   These tender points are located on the plantar surface of the foot along the medial or lateral aspects of the shaft of the fourth metatarsal or the medial aspect of the shaft of the fifth metatarsal. Pressure is applied in a cephalad direction and medially or laterally.

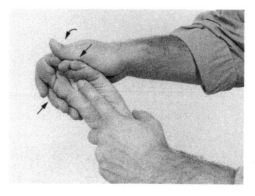

Position of Treatment   The patient is prone with the involved knee flexed and the dorsum of the foot resting on the therapist's thigh. The therapist grasps the foot from both sides and squeezes to cause inversion of the fourth and fifth metatarsals. Internal or external rotation is used to fine-tune the position.

References

1. Bogduk N, Tynan W, Wilson AS: The nerve supply of the human lumbar intervertebral discs, *J Anat* 132:39, 1981.
2. Brown CW: The natural history of thoracic disc degeneration, *Spine* (suppl): 1992.
3. Calais-Germain B: *Anatomy of movement*, Seattle, 1993, Eastland Press.
4. D'Ambrogio K: *Strain/counterstrain study guide*, rev ed, Palm Beach, 1991, Upledger Institute.
5. Deig D: *Positional release techniques*, Indianapolis, 1986, Broad Ripple Physical Therapy, self-published.
6. Donatelli RA, Walker R: Lower quarter evaluation: structural relationships and interdependence. In Donatelli RA, Wooden MJ, editors: *Orthopaedic physical therapy*, ed 2, New York, 1992, Churchill Livingstone.
7. Greenfield B: upper quarter evaluation: structural relationships and interdependence. In Donatelli RA, Wooden MJ, editors: *Orthopaedic physical therapy*, ed 2, New York, 1992, Churchill Livingstone.
8. Hoover HV: Functional Technic, *AAO Year Book* 47, 1958.
9. Jones LH: *Strain and counterstrain*, Newark, Ohio, 1981, American Academy of Osteopathy.
10. Kendall FP, McCreary EK: *Muscles: testing and function*, Baltimore, 1983, Williams & Wilkins.
11. Korr IM: Proprioceptors and somatic dysfunction, *J Am Osteopath Assoc* 74:638, 1975.
12. Levin SM: The icosohedron as the three-dimensional finite element in biomechanical support. Proceedings of the Society of General Systems Research on Mental Images, Values and Reality, Society of General Systems Research, St. Louis, May 1986.
13. Mennel JM: Trigger points in referred spinal pain. In Grieve GP, editor: *Modern manual therapy of the vertebral column*, New York, 1986, Churchill Livingstone.
14. Netter F: *Atlas of human anatomy*, Summit, NJ, 1989, Ciba-Geigy.
15. Ramirez MA, Haman J, Worth L: Low back pain: diagnosis by six newly discovered sacral tender points and treatment with counterstrain, *J Am Osteopath Assoc* 89:7, 1989.
16. Rosomoff HL, Fishbain DA, Goldberg M, Steele-Rosomoff R: Physical findings in patients with chronic intractable benign pain of the neck and/or back, *Pain* 37:279, 1989.
17. Roth GB: *Counterstrain: positional release therapy, study guide*, Toronto, 1991, Wellness Institute.
18. Schwartz HR: The use of counterstrain in an acutely ill in-hospital population, *J Am Osteopath Assoc*, 86:433, 1986.
19. Sutherland WG: The cranial bowl, *J Am Osteopath Assoc* 2:348, 1944.
20. Tiberio D, Gray GW: Kinematics and kinetics during gait. In Donatelli RA, Wooden MJ, editors: *Orthopaedic physical therapy*, ed 2, New York, 1992, Churchill Livingstone.
21. Travell JG, Simons DG: *Myofascial pain and dysfunction: the trigger point manual*, Baltimore, 1983, Williams & Wilkins.
22. Upledger JE: *Craniosacral therapy*, Seattle, 1983, Eastland Press.
23. Weiselfish S: *Manual therapy for the orthopedic and neurologic patient emphasizing strain and counterstrain technique*, Hartford, Conn, 1993, Regional Physical Therapy.

7

The Use of Positional Release Therapy in Clinical Practice

¶HOW TO INCORPORATE POSITIONAL RELEASE THERAPY WITH OTHER MODALITIES

Positional release therapy helps normalize inappropriate proprioceptive activity and promotes the release of muscle guarding and fascial tension, thus increasing soft tissue flexibility, improving joint mobility, decreasing pain, increasing circulation, and decreasing swelling. By using PRT, the patient's muscle, fascia, and articular components are structurally normalized to a point where the therapist can start to implement a functional rehabilitation program. It is essential to perform a thorough reevaluation at each visit. In most cases the patient's pain level will be dramatically reduced in the first few visits so that the patient can progress with cardiovascular fitness, strengthening, mobility, and range-of-motion exercises. Modalities may be used for pain management and swelling or to help promote soft-tissue healing. Positional release therapy may not be the primary treatment for all conditions, but it will help many patients overcome certain aspects of the dysfunction.

Based on the evaluation and determination of the cause of the dysfunction, other modalities may be introduced. In the case of persisting articular restriction, these may include manipulation, mobilization, or muscle energy. If the cranial structures are not fully corrected or the dural tube is under tension, cranial osteopathy or craniosacral therapy may be applied. With visceral or fascial involvement, the appropriate soft tissue technique is used. If the patient demonstrates muscle weakness, a strengthening program should be instituted. Frequently, massage and general exercise programs can further release tight, overused muscles, ease fascial tension, and help promote increased circulation. Modalities such as ice, heat, and electrical stimulation can aid in relaxing the patient and can help resolve inflammation, posttreatment soreness, and other reactions.

THE USE OF REALITY CHECKS

Reality checks are orthopedic and functional tests used to confirm various outcomes. These tests must be objective and measurable. The pain scale from 0 to 10 may be used (0 being no pain and 10 being the most severe) or a range-of-motion test (the patient lifts his arm over his head while the practitioner uses a goniometer to measure the range in degrees). Joint hypomobility tests (spinal or sacral spring tests) and functional tests (doing a deep squat or going up and down stairs) can also be used. If a patient has low back pain, the range of motion should be evaluated in each of the three planes. If it is found that there is pain at $^8/_{10}$ on left side bending and extension at ¼ range, these are two reality checks that can be used to confirm the outcome of treatment. Therefore when using PRT it is now possible to monitor left side bending and extension after treatment to see if there is a change in the pain level or range of motion. Thus it is important to find two or three objective measurements throughout the treatment program. It is also important to make the patient aware of these reality checks because this will be helpful in motivating the patient as changes occur.

HOW DO YOU COMMUNICATE WITH PATIENTS REGARDING POSITIONAL RELEASE THERAPY?

Communication is one of the most important aspects in dealing with the public. On the first visit, it is crucial that the subjective evaluation of the painful areas be recorded. It should also be noted whether the pain is constant, periodic, or occasional. Have the patients grade pain from 0 to 10, with 0 being no pain and 10 being the most severe. What do they expect to get from therapy? As health care providers, we must keep our patients focused on their own goals. Also, they must decide what they are prepared to do to obtain these goals. How will they know if they have obtained their goals? What reality checks will be used? It must be made clear to patients how their bodies will move and what they should feel. Some patients have no idea what wellness feels like. Each patient's expected outcome of therapy should be discussed and recorded by the practitioner to ensure that the goals will be met.

It is important to discuss the rationale of PRT. The patient must understand why a full-body evaluation is critical even when a specific site is so obviously painful. Men-

tion that either through various injuries sustained in the past or from the present injury, the tissues may have become injured and are in a shortened, tense position. This can result in the tissues being tender to the touch. If these tissues (muscles, ligaments, etc.) become short and tense, they will create joint stiffness and limit movement.

Patients will realize that trauma obtained in the past can result in accumulated restrictions throughout the body. To explain areas of dysfunction that are remote from the perceived symptoms, the analogy of a pulled garment, such as a sweater or blouse, can be used. This demonstrates that fascial restrictions, like fabric, can cause lines of tension to radiate from the source and thus cause strain in surrounding areas. (See Chapter 2, Fig. 2-4.)

Once the patient understands the purpose of the full-body evaluation, the therapist should proceed to explain what the patient can expect during and after the treatment session. It is suggested that the therapist find a tender point to demonstrate the PRT technique and gently bring the patient into and out of the position of comfort. This shows the patient that the tenderness will disappear in the position of comfort and demonstrates that the treatment is gentle and safe. It is important to explain that the patient may experience release phenomena consisting of pulsation, vibration, paresthesias, pain, or heat while in the position of comfort. These sensations will dissipate when a release in the soft tissues is completed. The patient should be informed that there should be a significant reduction in tenderness. The patient should be relaxed, more comfortable, and able to move more freely. During the 24 to 48 hours after the first treatment, approximately 40% of patients report some increased discomfort. Reassure the patient that this discomfort will disappear after a day or two and that an improvement in the original symptoms will be noticed. It is helpful to advise the patient that the discomfort may be felt directly in the area treated or that it may be felt elsewhere. For example, if the sacrum is treated, the patient may feel discomfort in the sacrum, neck, shoulder, or other areas of the body.

If these pretreatment discussions are omitted, the probability of future problems with the patient is extremely high. Thus it is necessary to prepare the patient and make sure that he is aware of the different sensations he may experience. When the practitioner clearly explains what is to be expected, the patient feels respected and included in the treatment program. He appreciates that the technique is gentle and that immediate results may be felt. The patient values the time taken, and this ensures satisfaction and confidence with both the practitioner and the rehabilitation program.

WHAT HAPPENS IF A TENDER POINT DOES NOT SHUT OFF?

Clinically, this has been found to be a rare occurrence. From our experience, when a therapist is unable to shut off a tender point, she must first establish if she is palpating the exact location of the tender point. Some points are close together. For example, the *anterior third lumbar,* which is on the lateral aspect of the anterior inferior iliac spine, is in close proximity to the tender point for the *gluteus minimus,* which is 1 cm lateral to the anterior inferior iliac spine. To treat an *anterior third lumbar,* the patient is placed into bilateral hip flexion of 90 degrees and side bent sharply away from the tender point side (p. 148). To treat a gluteus minimus, only the involved hip is flexed to approximately 130 degrees with 0 degrees of abduction and rotation (p. 152). In this situation, these two points are in close proximity, yet their treatments are different. It is essential that the practitioner know exactly which point is being treated.

Second, the practitioner may be on the desired point but the technique is not being performed properly, or palpation of the comfort zone has not been successfully attained to achieve the ideal position of relaxation. Standard procedure might call for only 90 degrees of flexion, but a particular patient may need 120 degrees of flexion to shut that point off. Therefore it is important that the *comfort zone* be carefully palpated and that the therapist be aware of the maximal tissue relaxation, using this as a guide to fine-tune the technique.

Third, are all the general rules being followed properly? Is the most severe tender point or area of greatest accumulation of tender points being treated first? Is the treatment being performed from proximal to distal? Maybe the point being treated will not shut off because there is another point that is dominant and must be treated before this one.

Fourth, there will be occasions when the desired point has been identified and the appropriate treatment is attempted, but for some reason it does not work. It is important to remember that "the patient is always right." The patient's body knows more about its needs than the therapist does, and it is vital to listen to what it tells you. The treatment positions have evolved from over 40 years of clinical experience and were developed by testing different positions on patients and finding which positions seemed to decrease the tenderness and relax the tissues. In most cases there will be a position that will shut the tender point off and relax the patient's tissues. (See the following section on conflicting points.) The therapist should start off with flexion and extension and determine which relaxes the tissues more. Then she should add rotation to the left and to the right. To which movement does the patient's body respond better? Next the therapist should add side bending to the left and right and then fine tune the position. As the therapist learns to dialogue with the tissues and gain experience through her hands, she will be able to develop new treatment positions for points that are not covered in this book.

If the tender point returns immediately after treatment, there may be a facilitated segment, suggesting that an inflammation or pathologic process is accentuating the sensitivity of the myofascial tissues and creating a secondary

tender point. The practitioner should be alert to this possibility if the tissues do not respond as expected. Further investigations or an appropriate referral may be required.

¶HOW DO YOU TREAT CONFLICTING POINTS?

A patient who has experienced a whiplash type of injury, for example, may have tender points in the anterior and posterior aspects of the neck. The practitioner may find that an attempt to treat the anterior lesion by flexing the patient's neck may cause the posterior pain or tenderness to intensify. This is a case of conflicting tender points and may be difficult to treat. This situation may warrant searching elsewhere in the body for an equally sensitive tender point. Treating another equally sensitive tender point remote from this area may cause one of the conflicting points to release, and treatment may then continue. If treatment of an equally sensitive tender point does not facilitate a change, the therapist should try other treatment modalities, such as craniosacral therapy, myofascial release, or muscle energy technique. It is important to remember that the patient must be comfortable and relaxed while being treated, and if there is any pain while being placed into the position of comfort, it is a contraindication to that particular treatment.

¶ANY SUGGESTIONS WHEN WORKING WITH OBESE PATIENTS?

The size of the patient must be considered. Assistive devices, such as a physioball or chair on which to rest the patient's legs, should be employed to prevent the therapist from bearing the weight. In some cases, an assistant may be helpful for the treatment. The therapist should never try to support the weight with only his hands or arms. He should bring the weight in close to his body and use the larger muscle groups, such as the trunk and legs, for support. It is important to be sure that the table is at an appropriate height to prevent injury to the therapist. The safety of the therapist must always remain a consideration. Specialized positioning tables, such as the one developed by one of us (Roth), may be of great value in reducing strain (see the Appendix).

With regard to palpation of tender points on obese people, a thorough grasp of anatomy is mandatory. Gently sink the fingers into the tissue, spreading some of the fat out of the way to locate the desired point. Palpation may be slightly more difficult and time consuming, but it is possible.

¶ANY FURTHER SUGGESTIONS WITH REGARD TO ERGONOMICS AND PROPER BODY MECHANICS?

Throughout the treatment section in this book, recommendations are made that will help the therapist ergonomically. The height of the practitioner, the size of the patient, and the height of the table may vary. It is imperative that the practitioner always remain in a comfortable treatment position. An adjustable table is ideal; however, a footstool can compensate for some differences. It is important to employ proper fulcrums and bear the weight properly without discomfort. The therapist should never try to support weight with outstretched hands or arms. The weight should be brought in as close to the therapist's body as possible and the larger muscles used for support. A large physioball or chair may be used to support the patient's legs. The ball or chair can be moved easily to assist the patient in side bending and rotation. Different-sized wedges, pillows, and chairs may be employed to support the patient's body weight. When using the hands to apply pressure, the wrists should be locked in extension, elbows extended, and shoulders placed directly over the hands when performing compression so that the larger muscle groups are used to deliver the force and not the hands.

In the event that a heavy body part requires lifting, the therapist should extend the elbows, lean back, and use her own body weight to create mechanical advantage.

¶Does Positional Release Therapy Specifically Treat Soft Tissue Damage?

Positional release therapy mainly treats *inappropriate proprioceptive activity* and fascial tension and thus decreases protective muscle spasm, increases strength, decreases swelling, increases circulation, and improves joint mobility. It removes many barriers to allow the body to use more of its resources to assist the healing process. If there is torn tissue, PRT may facilitate a better environment for healing, but the technique does not directly repair the tissue damage. The tissues require time to heal on their own or may require surgical intervention in rare cases.

According to Levin, neuromusculoskeletal dysfunction is a nonlinear event. This means that it is mediated by neural and electrochemical changes that require a minimal amount of time to develop (i.e., a sudden strain) and almost no time to resolve once a corrective intervention is applied. Linear processes, such as fractures, tears, and lacerations, require a substantial time interval for the healing process to effect a repair of the tissue damage. Positional release therapy is a nonlinear therapy and addresses the nonlinear aspect of the injury.

¶Can Positional Release Therapy Address Repetitive Strain Injuries?

The issue of repetitive strain injury (RSI), also referred to as *cumulative trauma disorder* (CTD), is in the forefront of industrial health care and is a subject of much speculation. Symptoms of pain, parasthesia, and weakness are associated with repetitive occupational activities and are seen in many industrial settings. These conditions appear to be associated with a combination of ergonomic and behavioral factors including sustained posture and poor body mechanics on the part of the employee. Repetitive motion and sustained posture on production lines within the manufacturing sector and clerical and technical occupations associated with the use of computer terminals are common factors causing high risk for CTD. Muscular, fascial, articular, and neural inflammation have been implicated as the sources of symptoms.

It is the opinion of the authors that symptoms often arise in a certain part of the body because of the complex interactions of the tissues. This is in response to an aberrant distribution of forces related to background centers of fixation. These areas of fixation (dysfunction) would result in compensatory hypermobility of structures in other areas of the body. These secondary areas would be subject to excessive motion and stretching of tissues (strain). This excessive motion, especially if repetitive, could lead to the microtrauma and the ensuing release of nociceptive chemical mediators associated with the production of pain. Depending on the pattern of compensation, certain activities may directly engage muscular tissues resulting in overstretching of these structures. This would lead to a myostatic reflex response of increased contraction, tissue ischemia, anaerobic metabolism, metabolic waste accumulation, and the release of pain producing chemical substances. Depending on the pattern of dysfunction, this reflex contraction may result in direct impingement of a nerve tract, leading to parasthesia and weakness.

Positional Release Therapy can help to address the complex pattern of symptoms associated with CTD by relieving the background myofascial dysfunction, which can set the stage for the onset of this disorder. It is important to emphasize that, with CTD or RSI as with any other clinical disorder, it is the dysfunction rather than the symptoms that must guide the therapeutic intervention. Postural education, proper ergonomics, job management, and preventative exercise, along with the appropriate application of therapeutic principles such as those presented in this text, can help to address this significant source of absenteeism, reduced productivity, and unnecessary drain on health care resources.

¶What Happens If You Are Unable to Locate Significant Tender Points and Yet the Patient Has Pain?

It is important to remember that we have listed more than 200 tender points. These are by no means all the tender points in the body, but these are the ones that are explained in detail, because they appear most consistently. If none of these points is found to be tender, it may be necessary to reevaluate the patient for tender points in other locations. In these cases, the general rules should be used to treat any new point that is found. If no tenderness is found, other systems may be screened (the craniosacral system, myofascial system, articular system, etc.), or a more thorough diagnostic workup or appropriate referral may be required to rule out possible pathology or infection.

WHAT HAPPENS IF PAIN OR OTHER SENSATIONS OCCUR DURING THE TREATMENT WHILE THE PATIENT IS IN A POSITION OF COMFORT?

If a patient complains of pain while the therapist is seeking a position of comfort, some tissue that is in dysfunction is being stressed and the patient should not be kept in this position. This is a contraindication to that position. If it is possible to get the patient into a position of comfort without pain but a pain, ache, or paresthesia develops while the patient is being treated, this is acceptable. It is often part of the release phenomena and will not last more than a few minutes. The patient may also feel heat, vibrations, pulsations, or an internal movement of the myofascial component. Upledger calls this unwinding. If any of these sensations occur, it is important to maintain the position of treatment until the symptoms subside and a release is felt. The patient may experience these various sensations spontaneously in different regions of the body throughout the treatment session. It is important to reassure the patient that these sensations are part of the release phenomena and will not continue after the release has been completed.

WHAT ACTIVITIES CAN THE PATIENT PERFORM AFTER A POSITIONAL RELEASE THERAPY TREATMENT SESSION?

Clinically it has been found that a cessation of *strenuous* activity for the next 24 to 48 hours is recommended. The body is still extremely sensitive, and the protective muscle spasm can easily return. The tissues may also be connected to a facilitated segment that may be vulnerable to reactivation and require time to resolve. The patient may benefit from heat, massage, gentle mobilization, "aquabics," and range-of-motion exercises, as well as cardiovascular exercises, such as treadmill, bicycle, or upper-body cycle. These forms of treatment help increase circulation, mobility, and flexibility; help decrease stiffness; and may alleviate posttreatment soreness, as long as the exercises are gentle and there is no strenuous component.

WHAT CAN PATIENTS DO ABOUT POSTTREATMENT SORENESS?

Posttreatment soreness usually lasts for approximately a day or two and can be somewhat relieved by gentle exercise and consuming water to assist the body in the elimination of accumulated metabolites such as histamines. Other techniques that encourage circulation, the efficient elimination of toxins, and mental and physical relaxation may be extremely valuable in minimizing posttreatment reactions. Hydrotherapy, in the form of ice and heat, whirlpool baths, contrast or epsom salt baths, and alternating hot and cold showers, has been effective in providing relief to many patients. Relaxation and breathing exercises can be taught to patients. The application of therapeutic modalities, such as ultrasound, interferential current, diathermy, and microcurrent, may be useful in treating possible reactions. In certain cases, over-the-counter analgesics may be necessary to help diminish the inflammatory process.

DO YOU OFFER ANY HOME PROGRAMS TO YOUR PATIENTS?

Yes. For example, if a patient has a psoas muscle that has been in spasm for several years and that does not fully release during the treatment session, the patient will be given home positional release exercises to further relax that muscle. A patient who keeps stressing a certain muscle because of the type of repetitive action or positioning at home or work could also benefit from a home program. These home PRT exercise programs are also highly recommended for those individuals who experience muscle tension because of traveling or muscle soreness resulting from exercise or athletics. Instead of doing stretching exercises, the patient will perform tissue-shortening exercises and then a series of other exercises to strengthen the muscles and mobilize the joints.

Home exercises also give some responsibility to patients for their own wellness. This can help focus their attention in a positive way on their bodies, instead of the negative association with pain. This combination can provide a valuable source of motivation for continuing the rehabilitation program and returning to normal activities more quickly. Patients who experience an acute flare-up will be able to help themselves until they can obtain medical attention, if necessary.

SUMMARY

This chapter has outlined several commonly asked questions that we have had to address during seminars. We have provided a quick reference guide for solutions to problems that therapists frequently encounter. This chapter has also addressed the importance of patient-practitioner communication and the need to identify treatment goals and expectations. Measures to reduce practitioner strain injury have been discussed, and specific ergonomic suggestions have been provided. In addition, we have outlined specific clinical challenges and methods to facilitate optimal results.

8

New Horizons

⁊Listening to the Tissues — Treating the Dysfunction

The goal of posititional release therapy (PRT) is to be able to identify the primary dysfunction and to direct therapy to the source of the dysfunction. The scanning evaluation is a useful tool that allows the practitioner to develop an objective basis for determining the primary tender points, which are an indication of the primary dysfunctions. This makes it possible to unravel the compensatory patterns that manifest as the presenting condition of the patient. Positional release therapy is one of a growing group of therapies that have evolved in recent years which recognize the inherent properties of organic tissue and attempt to work in harmony with them to restore optimal function.

The primary dysfunction is exemplified by fixation and loss of physiologic and non-physiologic motion. Fascial and neuromuscular mechanisms have been altered to resist deformation in the body's attempt to limit further destructive potential from ongoing or subsequent trauma. These changes result in the development of an area of persisting hypomobility. Over time, this area of relative fixation creates a new, abnormal center of motion in the body and thus induces overstretch, aberrant motion, and hypermobility in surrounding tissues. Pain rarely arises in tissue that is fixed. Putting a cast on a broken bone attests to this. It is the tissues and joints above and below the cast that become uncomfortable. Overstretched, strained, and hypermobile tissues around the area of fixation become inflamed and symptomatic. Thus, when we focus our attention on the area of symptoms in chronic conditions, we are usually dealing with secondary compensations and decompensation

indirectly related to the source of the condition. In acute cases, however, treatment directed to the area of symptoms is often at least partially appropriate.

The appearance of symptoms is a dilemma to the therapist. We listen to the history of the patient and would like to remove the discomfort or pain. This, for many of us, is our *raison d'être*. We live for the moment when we can come to the rescue and alleviate the suffering of our patients. We are, however, not always as successful as we would like to be. In many cases, when symptoms do abate, we would like to believe that it was through our efforts, but, if we are honest with ourselves, we must acknowledge that there may have been several other factors responsible for the apparent change. To be symptom oriented in practice is to be set up for failure. We are in constant doubt of our successes and failures because of the very nature of symptoms, which are the elusive and changeable outer manifestations of dysfunction.

Symptoms are variable, often self-limiting, and subjective by their very definition. However, the underlying dysfunction does not vary, is not self-limiting, and is totally objective by definition. Efficient diagnosis and appropriate therapeutic intervention directed toward the dysfunction should be the goal of therapy. For example, any firefighter will tell you that when confronted with flames, the extinguisher should be directed to the base of the flame, and if fuel is feeding the flames, this should be turned off first. This is an appropriate analogy to our clinical experience; much of the frustration and failure to which we have all been subject could be greatly reduced if we would adopt a similar attitude—that is, focus on the cause of the condition: the dysfunction.

The implications of the tensegrity model (see the Appendix, p. 246) from a clinical perspective are that all tissues share certain characteristics and that the artificial separation of tissue types and the application of particular therapeutic interventions to an isolated tissue may be counterproductive. Indeed, this model clearly confirms that all tissues are alike at the fundamental level and are interconnected in terms of the transmission of forces and possibly the conduction of electrochemical impulses. With regard to the use of PRT, we feel that any tissue may be implicated in the production of the apparent clinical presentation. Focusing on the dysfunction, no matter where it may appear, will liberate us from the tyranny of the elusive symptom and allow us to direct our energies to the cause of the condition rather than the effects.

ADAPTABILITY AND THE ROLE OF EXERCISE

Positional release therapy is a form of structural therapy that can help restore freedom of motion and functional integrity to the body. This is accomplished by releasing tension in the fascial, muscular, and articular systems. Positional release therapy removes barriers that restrict normal elasticity and tone of the tissues, thus allowing the patient to tolerate more easily, and benefit from, other aspects of the rehabilitation program.

The body has the ability to adapt to minor stresses but, as the number is increased, the body has less room to adapt until, a point is reached where the body cannot adapt any further. These stresses include environmental factors, emotional stress, and the effects of a sedentary lifestyle (i.e., lack of physical fitness).

A sedentary lifestyle tends to make a person more vulnerable to injury. Lack of physical activity is associated with reduced flexibility and strength within the musculoskeletal system and a deterioration of the posture. It is also associated with diminished cardiovascular fitness and disturbances in other systems (hormonal balance, glucose regulation, circulation, digestive function, etc.). Restriction of motion and joint fixation result in an uneven distribution of forces throughout the body during activities such as gait, exercise, lifting, and repetitive movements. This imbalance in forces may result in a reduced ability of the body to sustain injuries, creating a greater possibility for the development of dysfunction. Emotional stress, metabolic disturbances, and visceral pathophysiology mediated by a facilitated segment, may also feed into the pattern of dysfunction and further reduce the adaptability of the individual.

A complete rehabilitation program should include both *structural* and *functional* therapies. The goal of structural therapy is to restore symmetry and freedom of motion to the body. The goal of functional therapy is to develop strength, balance, and vitality within the tissues and restore optimal function within the context of the individual's occupation and activities of daily living. Structural therapy is a passive process, whereas functional rehabilitation, including specific exercise programs, requires the active participation and cooperation of the patient.

Most people acknowledge the importance of exercise as part of a program to restore function after an injury and to maintain optimal health. Many, however, find it difficult to motivate themselves to follow through on this aspect of their rehabilitation program. The active component of therapy is often introduced before structural restoration has occurred, and these patients frequently experience an aggravation of their symptoms. This is a common mistake in therapy and is a significant reason for failure of the rehabilitation process. Positional release therapy and other structural therapies are necessary to prepare the tissues so that they can tolerate exercise. It may be difficult to motivate patients to incorporate exercise into their lives. However, education and diligence in formulating programs that are achievable and enjoyable are keys to overcoming this obstacle.

A sedentary individual may also lack the coordination necessary to perform certain activities in a smooth and efficient manner. This can be a factor leading to an increased susceptibility to injury. An athletic individual, on the other hand, may have a much greater tolerance to exercise. The active program must therefore be matched to the patient's fitness level: gradual and progressive in the case of the sedentary person and challenging enough to motivate the athlete and the physically fit subject.

A person who is flexible, strong, coordinated, and in a general state of optimal health is less vulnerable to the development of dysfunction as the result of injuries. Such a person may, indeed, be less likely to be injured in the first place because of a heightened state of mental alertness and a higher level of physical coordination. An individual who is fit has a greater adaptable range in the ability to compensate for the effects of an injury and therefore is more likely to recover quickly and has a reduced tendency to have persisting dysfunction.

Although PRT is a passive therapeutic intervention, it is possible to incorporate it into the active part of the program. Certain PRT treatments can be adapted to be performed by the patient, especially in cases where repetitive trauma (RSI) may be unavoidable in the patient's occupation or lifestyle. This aspect of the program can be introduced once the major dysfunctions have been addressed. These exercises may be gradually augmented by progressive mobility exercises and strengthening regimens.

DEVELOPING THE ART AND SCIENCE OF POSITIONAL RELEASE THERAPY

A new paradigm is emerging in our understanding of the structure and function of the musculoskeletal system and how this relates to the etiology and resolution of dysfunction. The underlying nature of the body tissues, both under normal conditions and as they express dysfunction, reflect an inherent wisdom and order beyond our inadequate attempts to force them into our models or belief systems.

We are beginning to appreciate the dynamic, self-regulating, and interdependent nature of all living tissue. This new paradigm represents an acknowledgment of the *intrinsic* wisdom of the body and its inherent, self-healing potential. As our understanding of the nature of dysfunction has evolved, we are adapting our therapies into greater congruency with this evolving reality.

Several clinicians and researchers have been instrumental in revealing the nature of the human body and directing us to open a dialogue with the tissues in order to access these truths. Instead of forcing the patient's body into compliance, when it resists, we now have several powerful techniques that work in harmony with the natural, self-corrective processes inherent in the tissues. These methods have been gradually gaining acceptance in many branches of physical medicine because of their effectiveness and nontraumatic nature.

Positional release therapy has the potential to address many resistant cases of musculoskeletal dysfunction. The use of the tender points affords it a high degree of diagnostic accuracy and predictability. Achieving the comfort zone is readily discernible by the practitioner and the patient, and attention to the release process will ensure consistent results.

As with any skill, diligent practice will gradually lead to proficiency. We urge the practitioner to learn the scanning evaluation, which when mastered can be completed in a few minutes. This will reveal the hidden truth behind the presenting symptoms. Practicing the treatment positions and developing good body mechanics take time. The positive response of your patients will, we hope, motivate your persistence in developing these skills.

In conclusion, we recommend that this text be used as a handy desk reference. The scanning evaluation can be copied and used for each patient, and the tender point body charts can be copied and laminated for quick reference. The treatment section of the book can be readily referred to by flipping it open to the appropriate page and following the directions for the dominant tender points. We urge you to wear this book out. By the time that occurs, you may find that you no longer need to refer to it. For those interested in hands-on instruction and the development of advanced skills, the authors present seminars internationally. For information about these programs please contact the authors.

Appendix

Positional Release Therapy Scanning Evaluation

Patient's name:_____ Practitioner: _____

Dates: 1_____   2_____   3_____   4_____   5_____

● - Extremely sensitive   ◑ - Very sensitive   ◐ - Moderately sensitive   ○ - No tenderness

\ - Right   / - Left   + - Most sensitive   Ȯ - Treatment

I.   Cranium (p. 45)

1. OM	○○○○○	6. DG	○○○○○	11. NAS	○○○○○	16. AT	○○○○○
2. OCC	○○○○○	7. MPT	○○○○○	12. SO	○○○○○	17. PT	○○○○○
3. PSB	○○○○○	8. LPT	○○○○○	13. FR	○○○○○	18. TPA	○○○○○
4. LAM	○○○○○	9. MAS	○○○○○	14. SAG	○○○○○	19. TPP	○○○○○
5. SH	○○○○○	10. MAX	○○○○○	15. LSB	○○○○○	_____	○○○○○

II.   Anterior, Medial, Lateral Cervical Spine (p. 66)

20. AC1	○○○○○	23. AC4	○○○○○	26. AC7	○○○○○	29. LC1	○○○○○
21. AC2	○○○○○	24. AC5	○○○○○	27. AC8	○○○○○	30. LC__	○○○○○
22. AC3	○○○○○	25. AC6	○○○○○	28. AMC	○○○○○	30. LC__	○○○○○

III.   Posterior Cervical Spine (p. 78)

31. PC1-F	○○○○○	34. PC3	○○○○○	37. PC6	○○○○○	_____	○○○○○
32. PC1-E	○○○○○	35. PC4	○○○○○	38. PC7	○○○○○	_____	○○○○○
33. PC2	○○○○○	36. PC5	○○○○○	39. PC8	○○○○○	_____	○○○○○

IV.   Anterior Thoracic Spine (p. 86)

40. AT1	○○○○○	43. AT4	○○○○○	46. AT7	○○○○○	49. AT10	○○○○○
41. AT2	○○○○○	44. AT5	○○○○○	47. AT8	○○○○○	50. AT11	○○○○○
42. AT3	○○○○○	45. AT6	○○○○○	48. AT9	○○○○○	51. AT12	○○○○○

V.   Anterior and Medial Ribs (p. 91)

52. AR1	○○○○○	57. AR6	○○○○○	62. MR3	○○○○○	67. MR8	○○○○○
53. AR2	○○○○○	58. AR7	○○○○○	63. MR4	○○○○○	68. MR 9	○○○○○
54. AR3	○○○○○	59. AR8	○○○○○	64. MR5	○○○○○	69. MR10	○○○○○
55. AR4	○○○○○	60. AR9	○○○○○	65. MR6	○○○○○	_____	○○○○○
56. AR5	○○○○○	61. AR10	○○○○○	66. MR7	○○○○○	_____	○○○○○

VI.   Anterior Lumbar Spine (p. 145)

130. AL1	○○○○○	132. AL2	○○○○○	134. AL4	○○○○○	_____	○○○○○
131. ABL2	○○○○○	133. AL3	○○○○○	135. AL5	○○○○○	_____	○○○○○

VII.   Anterior Pelvis & Hip (p. 151)

136. IL	○○○○○	138. SAR	○○○○○	140. SPB	○○○○○	142. LPB	○○○○○
137. GMI	○○○○○	139. TFL	○○○○○	141. IPB	○○○○○	143. ADD	○○○○○

VIII.   Knee (p. 183)

168. PAT	○○○○○	171. LK	○○○○○	174. PES	○○○○○	177. POP	○○○○○
169. PTE	○○○○○	172. MH	○○○○○	175. ACL	○○○○○	_____	○○○○○
170. MK	○○○○○	173. LH	○○○○○	176. PCL	○○○○○	_____	○○○○○

IX. Ankle (p. 194)

178. MAN	○○○○○	181. TAL	○○○○○	184. FDL	○○○○○	187. EDL	○○○○○
179. LAN	○○○○○	182. PAN	○○○○○	185. TBA	○○○○○	_____	○○○○○
180. AAN	○○○○○	183. TBP	○○○○○	186. PER	○○○○○	_____	○○○○○

X. Foot (p. 205)

188. MCA	○○○○○	194. PNV	○○○○○	200. PCN3	○○○○○	206. PMT1	○○○○○
189. LCA	○○○○○	195. DCN1	○○○○○	201. DMT1	○○○○○	207. PMT2	○○○○○
190. PCA	○○○○○	196. DCN2	○○○○○	202. DMT2	○○○○○	208. PMT3	○○○○○
191. DCB	○○○○○	197. DCN3	○○○○○	203. DMT3	○○○○○	209. PMT4	○○○○○
192. PCB	○○○○○	198. PCN1	○○○○○	204. DMT4	○○○○○	210. PMT5	○○○○○
193. DNV	○○○○○	199. PCN2	○○○○○	205. DMT5	○○○○○	_____	○○○○○

XI. Shoulder (p. 106)

94. TRA	○○○○○	99. SUB	○○○○○	104. PMI	○○○○○	109. ISS	○○○○○
95. SCL	○○○○○	100. SER	○○○○○	105. LD	○○○○○	110. ISM	○○○○○
96. AAC	○○○○○	101. MHU	○○○○○	106. PAC	○○○○○	111. ISI	○○○○○
97. SSL	○○○○○	102. BSH	○○○○○	107. SSM	○○○○○	112. TMA	○○○○○
98. BLH	○○○○○	103. PMA	○○○○○	108. MSC	○○○○○	113. TMI	○○○○○

XII. Elbow (p. 127)

114. LEP	○○○○○	116. RHS	○○○○○	118. MCD	○○○○○	120. MOL	○○○○○
115. MEP	○○○○○	117. RHP	○○○○○	119. LCD	○○○○○	121. LOL	○○○○○

XIII. Wrist & Hand (p. 134)

122. CFT	○○○○○	124. PWR	○○○○○	126. CM1	○○○○○	128. DIN	○○○○○
123. CET	○○○○○	125. DWR	○○○○○	127. PIN	○○○○○	129. IP	○○○○○

XIV. Posterior Thoracic Spine (p. 96)

70. PT1	○○○○○	73. PT4	○○○○○	76. PT7	○○○○○	79. PT10	○○○○○
71. PT2	○○○○○	74. PT5	○○○○○	77. PT8	○○○○○	80. PT11	○○○○○
72. PT3	○○○○○	75. PT6	○○○○○	78. PT9	○○○○○	81. PT12	○○○○○

XV. Posterior Ribs (p. 101)

82. PR1	○○○○○	85. PR4	○○○○○	88. PR7	○○○○○	91. PR10	○○○○○
83. PR2	○○○○○	86. PR5	○○○○○	89. PR8	○○○○○	92. PR11	○○○○○
84. PR3	○○○○○	87. PR6	○○○○○	90. PR9	○○○○○	93. PR12	○○○○○

XVI. Posterior Lumbar Spine (p. 160)

144. PL1	○○○○○	147. PL4	○○○○○	150. PL3-I	○○○○○	153. LPL5	○○○○○
145. PL2	○○○○○	148. PL5	○○○○○	151. PL4-I	○○○○○	_____	○○○○○
146. PL3	○○○○○	149. QL	○○○○○	152. UPL5	○○○○○	_____	○○○○○

XVII. Posterior Pelvis & Hip (p. 167)

154. SSI	○○○○○	156. ISI	○○○○○	158. PRM	○○○○○	160. GME	○○○○○
155. MSI	○○○○○	157. GEM	○○○○○	159. PRL	○○○○○	161. ITB	○○○○○

XVIII. Posterior Sacrum (p. 175)

162. PS1	○○○○○	164. PS3	○○○○○	166. PS5	○○○○○	_____	○○○○○
163. PS2	○○○○○	165. PS4	○○○○○	167. COX	○○○○○	_____	○○○○○

TENDER POINT BODY CHARTS

Spine/Pelvis/Rib Tender Points

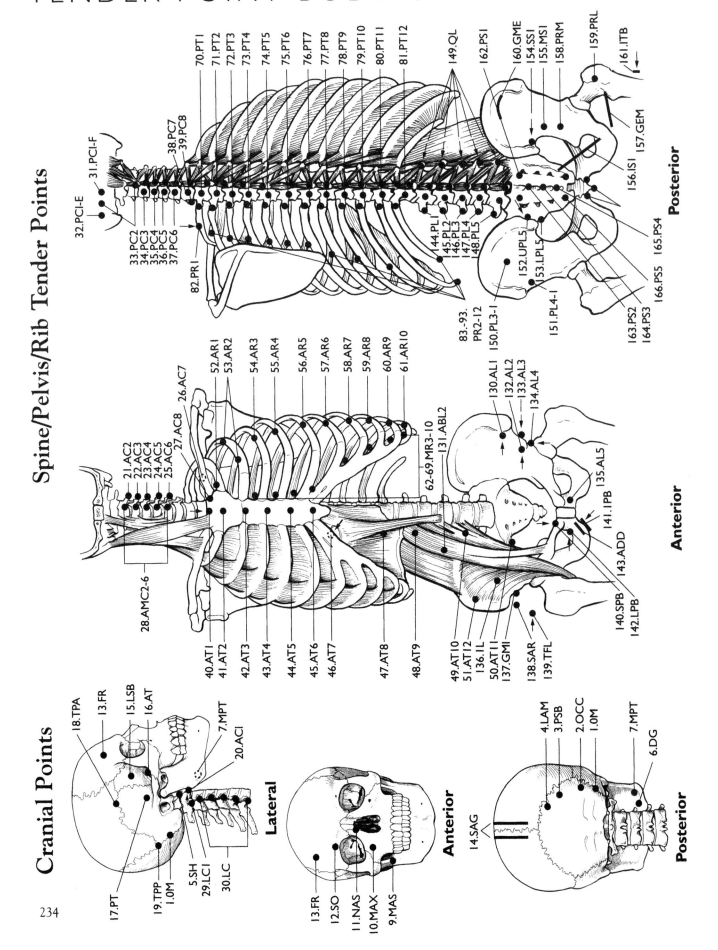

Posterior

70.PT1
71.PT2
72.PT3
73.PT4
74.PT5
75.PT6
76.PT7
77.PT8
78.PT9
79.PT10
80.PT11
81.PT12
149.QL
162.PS1
160.GME
154.SS1
155.MS1
158.PRM
159.PRL
161.ITB
157.GEM
156.ISI
32.PCI-E
31.PCI-F
38.PC7
39.PC8
33.PC2
34.PC3
35.PC4
36.PC5
37.PC6
82.PR1
144.PL1
145.PL2
146.PL3
147.PL4
148.PL5
152.UPL5
153.LPL5
151.PL4-I
150.PL3-I
83.-93.PR2-12
163.PS2
164.PS3
166.PS5
165.PS4

Anterior

52.AR1
53.AR2
54.AR3
55.AR4
56.AR5
57.AR6
58.AR7
59.AR8
60.AR9
61.AR10
26.AC7
27.AC8
21.AC2
22.AC3
23.AC4
24.AC5
25.AC6
62-69.MR3-10
131.ABL2
130.AL1
132.AL2
133.AL3
134.AL4
135.AL5
141.IPB
143.ADD
140.SPB
142.LPB
138.SAR
139.TFL
137.GMI
136.IL
50.AT11
51.AT12
49.AT10
48.AT9
47.AT8
46.AT7
45.AT6
44.AT5
43.AT4
42.AT3
41.AT2
40.AT1
28.AMC2-6

Cranial Points

18.TPA
13.FR
15.LSB
16.AT
7.MPT
20.ACI
17.PT
19.TPP
1.0M
5.SH
29.LCI
30.LC

Lateral

Anterior

13.FR
12.SO
11.NAS
10.MAX
9.MAS

Posterior

4.LAM
3.PSB
2.OCC
1.0M
7.MPT
6.DG
14.SAG

234

Shoulder Tender Points

94.TRA
95.SCL
96.AAC
104.PMI
102.BSH
98.BLH
103.PMA
100.SER

Anterior

108.MSC

Posterior

107.SSM
106.PAC
97.SSL
109.ISS
113.TMI
110.ISM
111.ISI
112.TMA
105.LD

Elbow/Wrist/Hand Tender Points

114.LEP
118.MCD
119.LCD
124.PWR
127.PIN

115.MEP
116.RHS
117.RHP
126.CMI
129.IP

Palmar

120.MOL
121.LOL
125.DWR
128.DIN

Dorsal

Ankle/Foot Tender Points

179.LAN

Lateral

189.LCA

188.MCA
181.TAL
178.MAN

Medial

180.AAN
193.DNV
195-197. DCN1,2,3
201, 202. DMT1,2
203, 204. DMT3,4
191.DCB
204,205. DMT4,5

Dorsal

206, 207. PMT1,2
198-200. PCN1,2,3
194.PNV
190.PCA
182.PAN
207,208.PMT2,3
209,210. PMT4,5
192.PCB

Plantar

Knee Tender Points

172.MH
177.POP
182.PAN
184.FDL

175.ACL
176.PCL
173.LH
183.TBP

Posterior

168.PAT
171.LK
185.TBA
187.EDL
186.PER

170.MK
169.PTE
174.PES

Anterior

235

⌐Anatomy/Positional Release Therapy Cross-Reference

Muscles are listed by name only; other tissues are specified (bone, joint, etc.).

Anatomic Reference	Positional Release Therapy Reference	Page
Acromioclavicular joint	AAC, PAC	108, 118
Adductor hallucis	PMT1	217
Adductors	ADD	158
Anconeus	LOL, MOL	132
Anterior cruciate ligament	ACL	190
Biceps	BLH, BSH	110, 114
Brachialis	LCD, MCD	131
Coccygeus	ISI, COX	169, 180
Common extensor tendon	CET	135
Common flexor tendon	CFT	134
Coracoacromial ligament	AAC	108
Coronal suture	FR	57
Cuboid (bone)	DCB, PCB	208, 209
Cuneiform (bones)	DCN 1-3, PCN 1-3	212, 213
Deltoid anterior	AAC	108
Deltoid ligament	MAN	194
Diaphragm	AT7-9	88
Digastric	DG	50
Dorsal calcaneocuboid ligament	DCB	208
Dorsal cuneounavicular ligament	DCN 1-3	212
Dorsal interossei	DIN, DMT2,3, DMT4,5	140, 215, 216
Extensor digitorum longus	AAN, EDL	
	DMT2,3, DMT4,5	196, 203, 215, 216
Extensor hallucis longus	AAN, DMT1	196, 214
Flexor digiti minimi brevis	PMT4,5	219
Flexor digitorum brevis	PCA, DMT2,3, DMT4,5	207, 215, 216
Flexor digitorum longus	FDL	200
Flexor pollicis brevis	CM1	138
Frontal bone	FR	57
Frontonasal joint	SO	56
Gastrocnemius	PAN	198
Gemelli	GEM	170
Glenohumeral ligaments	MHU	113
Gluteus medius	GME, SSI	172, 167
Gluteus minimus	GMI, MSI	152, 168
Hamstrings, lateral	LH	188
Hamstrings, medial	MH	187
Iliacus	IL, AL1	151, 145
Iliococcygeus	IPB, LPL5	156, 165
Iliopsoas	AL2-5, LPL5	147, 165
Iliotibial band	ITB	173
Infraspinatus	ISS, ISM, ISI	121, 122, 123
Intercostal, external	MR3-10	94
Intercostal, internal	AT1-6, AR3-10	86, 87, 93
Interphalangeal joints	IP	141
Interspinalis, cervical	PC3-7	81, 82
Interspinalis, lumbar	PL1-5	160
Interspinalis, thoracic	PT1-12	96
Lambdoid suture	LAM, OCC	48, 46
Lateral collateral ligament	LK	186

Anatomic Reference	Positional Release Therapy Reference	Page
Lateral pterygoid	LPT	52
Latissimus dorsi	LD	117
Levator ani	PS1-5	175
Levator costorum	PC8, PR1-12	83, 101
Levator scapula	MSC	120
Longus capitis	AC3-5	68
Longus colli	AC2-6, AMC	67, 74
Lumbricals (foot)	PMT2,3	218
Masseter	MAS	53
Maxilla (bone)	MAX	54
Medial collateral ligament	MK	185
Medial pterygoid	MPT	51
Metacorpophalangeal joints	PIN, DIN	139, 140
Metatarsal (bones)	DMT, PMT	214, 217
Multifidus, cervical	PC3-7	81
Multifidus, lumbar	PL1-5, PL3, PL4-I, UPL5	160, 162, 163, 164
Multifidus, thoracic	PT1-12	96
Nasal bones	NAS, SO	55, 56
Navicular (bone)	DNV, PNV	210, 211
Obliquus capitis superior	PC1-E	79
Obturator externus	LPB	157
Occipital bone	OCC, LAM	46, 48
Occipitomastoid suture	OM	45
Opponens pollicis	CM1	138
Palmar interossei	PIN	139
Patellar retinaculum	PAT	183
Patellar tendon	PTE	184
Pectineus	LPB	157
Pectoralis major	PMA	115
Pectoralis minor	PMI	116
Peroneus	LAN, PER	195, 202
Peroneus tertius	DMT4,5	216
Piriformis	PRM, PRL	171
Plantar calcaneocuboid ligament	PCB	209
Plantar calcaneonavicular ligament	PNV	211
Plantar cuneonavicular ligament	PCN	213
Popliteus	POP	192
Posterior cruciate ligament	PCL	191
Pronator teres	RHP	130
Psoas	AT10-12, ABL2	89, 146
Pubococcygeus	COX, SPB	180, 155
Quadratus femoris	GEM	170
Quadratus lumborum	AT12, QL, PL3-I, PL4-I, PT10-12, UPL5, PR11, 12	89, 161, 162, 163, 99, 164, 103
Quadratus plantae	PCA	207
Quadriceps femoris	PAT, PTE	183, 184
Rectus capitis anterior	AC1, PC1-F	66, 78
Rectus capitis lateralis	LC1	75
Rectus capitis posterior	PC2	80
Rhomboid	MSC	120
Rotatores, cervical	PC3-7	81
Rotatores, lumbar	PL1-5, PL3,PL4-I, UPL5	160, 162, 163, 164
Rotatores, thoracic	PT1-12	96
Sacroiliac ligaments	UPL5, LPL5	164, 165

Anatomic Reference	Positional Release Therapy Reference	Page
Sacrospinous ligament	COX	180
Sacrotuberous ligament	COX, ISI	180, 169
Sagittal suture	SAG	58
Sartorius	SAR	153
Scalenus anterior	AC4-6	69
Scalenus medius	LC2-6, AR1	76, 91
Scalenus posterior	AR2, PR1	92, 101
Serratus anterior	SER	112
Soleus	PAN	198
Sphenobasilar suture	PSB, LSB	47, 59
Sternocleidomastoid	AC7	72
Sternothyroid	AT1	86
Stylohyoid	SH	49
Subclavius	SCL	107
Subscapularis	SUB	111
Supinator	RHS	129
Supraspinatus	SSM, SSL	119, 109
Talocalcaneal joint	MCA, LCA, PCA	205, 206, 207
Talofibular ligament	LAN	195
Talonavicular ligament	DNV	210
Temporalis	MAS, AT, PT	53, 60, 61
Temporomandibular joint	DG, MPT, LPT, MAS, MAX	50, 51, 52, 53, 54
Temporoparietal joint	TPA, TPP	62, 63
Tensor fascia lata	TFL	154
Tentorium cerebelli	OM	45
Teres major	TMA	124
Teres minor	TMI	125
Tibialis anterior	TAL, TBA	197, 201
Tibialis posterior	TBP	199
Transversus thoracis	MR3-10	94
Trapezius	TRA	106
Triceps	LOL, MOL	132
Wrist extensors	DWR	137
Wrist flexors	PWR	136
Zygomatic bone	AT, PT	60, 61

¶ STRAIN/COUNTERSTRAIN/POSITIONAL RELEASE THERAPY CROSS-REFERENCE

Strain/Counterstrain Terminology	Positional Release Therapy Terminology	Page
Abdominal second lumbar (Ab2L)	Abdominal second lumbar (ABL2)	146
Adductors (ADD)	Adductors (ADD)	158
Anterior acromioclavicular (AAC)	Anterior acromioclavicular (AAC)	108
Anterior cruciate ligament (ACL)	Anterior cruciate ligament (ACL)	190
Anterior eighth cervical (A8C)	Anterior eighth cervical (AC8)	73
Anterior eighth thoracic (A8T)	Anterior eighth thoracic (AT8)	88
Anterior eleventh thoracic (A11T)	Anterior eleventh thoracic (AT11)	89
Anterior fifth cervical (A5C)	Anterior fifth cervical (AC5)	70
Anterior fifth lumbar (A5L)	Anterior fifth lumbar (AL5)	149
Anterior fifth thoracic (A5T)	Anterior fifth thoracic (AT5)	87
Anterior first cervical (A1C)	Anterior first cervical (AC1)	66
Anterior first lumbar (A1L)	Anterior first lumbar (AL1)	145
Anterior first rib (A1R)	Anterior first rib (AR1)	91
Anterior first thoracic (A1T)	Anterior first thoracic (AT1)	86
Anterior fourth cervical (A4C)	Anterior fourth cervical (AC4)	69
Anterior fourth lumbar (A4L)	Anterior fourth lumbar (AL4)	148
Anterior fourth thoracic (A4T)	Anterior fourth thoracic (AT4)	87
Anterior lateral trochanter (ALT)	Sartorius (SAR)*	153
Anterior medial trochanter (AMT)	Gluteus minimus (GMI)*	152
Anterior ninth thoracic (A9T)	Anterior ninth thoracic (AT9)	88
Anterior second cervical (A2C)	Anterior second cervical (AC2)	67
Anterior second lumbar (A2L)	Anterior second lumbar (AL2)	147
Anterior second rib (A2R)	Anterior second rib (AR2)	92
Anterior second thoracic (A2T)	Anterior second thoracic (AT2)	86
Anterior seventh cervical (A7C)	Anterior seventh cervical (AC7)	72
Anterior seventh thoracic (A7T)	Anterior seventh thoracic (AT7)	88
Anterior sixth cervical (A6C)	Anterior sixth cervical (AC6)	71
Anterior sixth thoracic (A6T)	Anterior sixth thoracic (AT6)	87
Anterior tenth thoracic (A10T)	Anterior tenth thoracic (AT10)	89
Anterior third cervical (A3C)	Anterior third cervical (AC3)	68
Anterior third lumbar (A3L)	Anterior third lumbar (AL3)	148
Anterior third thoracic (A3T)	Anterior third thoracic (AT3)	86
Anterior third to sixth rib (A3R-A6R)	Anterolateral third to tenth rib (AR3-10)*	93
Anterior twelfth thoracic (A12T)	Anterior twelfth thoracic (AT12)	89
Bursa (BUR)	Supraspinatus lateral (SSL)*	109
Coccyx	Coccyx (COX)	180
Coronal (C)	Sagittal suture (SAG)*	58
Cuboid (CUB)	Plantar cuboid (PCB)*	209
Dorsal cuboid (DCU)	Dorsal cuboid (DCB)*	208
Dorsal fourth, fifth metatarsal (DM4,5)	Dorsal fourth, fifth metatarsal (DMT4,5)	216
Dorsal metatarsal (DM)	Dorsal first metatarsal (DMT1)*	214
Dorsal metatarsal (DM)	Dorsal second, third metatarsal (DMT2,3)	215
Dorsal wrist (DWR)	Dorsal wrist (DWR)	137
Elevated first rib	Posterior first rib (PR1)*	101
Elevated second to sixth ribs	Posterior second to tenth ribs (PR2-10)*	102
Extension ankle (EXA)	Posterior ankle (PAN)*	198
Extension carpometacarpal (ECM)	Dorsal interossei (DIN)*	140
First carpometacarpal (CMI)	First carpometacarpal (CM1)	138
Flexed ankle (FAN)	Anterior ankle (AAN)*	196
Flexion calcaneus (FCA)	Plantar calcaneus (PCA)*	207
Flexion medial calcaneus (FMC)	Tibialis posterior (TBP)*	199

Strain/Counterstrain Terminology	Positional Release Therapy Terminology	Page
Frontal (F)	Frontal (FR)*	57
Frozen Shoulder (FSH)	Medial humerus (MHU)*	113
Gluteus medius (GM)	Gluteus medius (GME)*	172
Gluteus minimus (GMI)	Tensor fascia lata (TFL)*	154
High flareout SI (HFO-SI)	Inferior sacroiliac (ISI)*	169
High ilium-sacroiliac (HISI)	Superior sacroiliac (SSI)*	167
High navicular (H.NAV)	Dorsal navicular (DNV)*	210
Iliacus (IL)	Iliacus (IL)	151
Infraorbital (IO)	Maxilla (MAX)*	54
Inguinal ligament (ING)	Lateral pubis (LPB)*	157
Inion	Posterior first cervical, flexion (PC1-F)*	78
Interossei (INT)	Palmar interossei (PIN)*	139
Interspace rib (4 Int-6 Int)	Medial third to tenth rib (MR3-10)*	94
Lambdoid (L)	Lambda (LAM)*	48
Lateral (1C)	Lateral first cervical (LC1)	75
Lateral ankle (LAN)	Lateral ankle (LAN)	195
Lateral ankle (LAN)	Peroneus (PER)*	202
Lateral calcaneus (LCA)	Lateral calcaneus (LCA)	206
Lateral canthus (LC)	Anterior temporalis (AT)*	60
Lateral epicondyle (LEP)	Lateral epicondyle (LEP)	127
Lateral hamstring (LH)	Lateral hamstring (LH)	188
Lateral/medial coronoid (LCD/MCD)	Lateral/medial coronoid (LCD/MCD)	131
Lateral meniscus (LM)	Lateral knee (LK)*	186
Lateral olecranon (LOL)	Lateral olecranon (LOL)	132
Lateral trochanter (LT)	Iliotibial band (ITB)*	173
Latissimus dorsi (LD)	Latissimus dorsi (LD)	117
Long head of biceps (LH)	Biceps long head (BLH)*	110
Low ilium-flareout (LIFO)	Inferior pubis (IPB)*	156
Low ilium-sacroiliac (LISI)	Superior pubis (SPB)*	155
Lower pole fifth lumbar (LP5L)	Lower posterior fifth lumbar (LPL5)*	165
LTS2	Infraspinatus superior (ISS)*	121
Masseter (M)	Masseter (MAS)*	53
Medial ankle (MAN)	Medial ankle (MAN)	194
Medial ankle (MAN)	Tibialis anterior (TBA)*	201
Medial calcaneus (MCA)	Medial calcaneus (MCA)	205
Medial coracoid (MC)	Pectoralis minor (PMI)*	116
Medial epicondyle (MEP)	Medial epicondyle (MEP)	128
Medial hamstring (MH)	Medial hamstring (MH)	187
Medial meniscus (MM)	Medial knee (MK)*	185
Medial olecranon (MOL)	Medial olecranon (MOL)	132
Metatarsal	Plantar metatarsal (PMT1-5)*	217
Midpole sacroiliac (MPSI)	Middle sacroiliac (MSI)*	168
MTS2	Medial scapula (MSC)**	120
Nasal (N)	Nasal (NAS)*	55
Navicular (NAV)	Plantar navicular (PNV)*	211
Occipitomastoid (OM)	Occipitomastoid (OM)	45
Patella (PAT)	Patella (PAT)	183
Patellar tendon (PTE)	Patellar tendon (PTE)	184
Pes anserinus (PES)	Pes anserinus (PES)	189
Piriformis (PIR)	Piriformis medial (PRM)*	171
Point on spine (POS)	Infraspinatus middle (ISM)*	122
Posterior acromioclavicular (PAC)	Posterior acromioclavicular (PAC)	118
Posterior auricular (PA)	Temporoparietal, post. (TPP)*	63
Posterior cruciate ligament (PCR)	Posterior cruciate ligament (PCL)*	191

Strain/Counterstrain Terminology	Positional Release Therapy Terminology	Page
Posterior eighth cervical (P8C)	Posterior eighth cervical (PC8)	83
Posterior fifth to seventh cervical (P5C, P6C, P7C)	Posterior fifth to seventh cervical (PC5-7)	82
Posterior first cervical (P1C)	Posterior first cervical, ext. (PC1-E)*	79
Posterior first, second lumbar (P1-2L)	Posterior first to fifth lumbar (PL1-5)**	160
Posterior first, second thoracic (P1-2T)	Posterior first, second thoracic (PT1-2)	96
Posterior fourth cervical (P4C)	Posterior fourth cervical (PC4)	82
Posterior fourth lumbar (P4L)	Posterior fourth lumbar, iliac (PL4-I)*	163
Posterior medial trochanter (PMT)	Gemelli (GEM)*	170
Posterior occipital (PO)	Occipital (OCC)*	46
Posterior sacrum 1 (PS1)	Posterior sacrum 1 (PS1)	175
Posterior sacrum 2 (PS2)	Posterior sacrum 2 (PS2)	176
Posterior sacrum 3 (PS3)	Posterior sacrum 3 (PS3)	177
Posterior sacrum 4 (PS4)	Posterior sacrum 4 (PS4)	178
Posterior sacrum 5 (PS5)	Posterior sacrum 5 (PS5)	179
Posterior second cervical (P2C)	Posterior second cervical (PC2)	80
Posterior sixth to ninth thoracic (P6-9T)	Posterior sixth to ninth thoracic (PT6-9)	98
Posterior tenth to twelfth thoracic (P10-12T)	Posterior tenth to twelfth thoracic (PT10-12)	99
Posterior third cervical (P3C)	Posterior third cervical (PC3)	81
Posterior third lumbar (P3L)	Posterior third lumbar, iliac (PL3-I)*	162
Posterior third to fifth thoracic (P3-5T)	Posterior third to fifth thoracic (PT3-5)	97
Posterolateral trochanter (PLT)	Piriformis lateral (PRL)*	171
Radial head (RAD)	Radial head pronator (RHP)*	130
Radial head (RAD)	Radial head supinator (RHS)*	129
Short head of biceps (SH)	Biceps short head (BSH)*	114
Sphenobasilar (SB)	Posterior sphenobasilar (PSB)*	47
Sphenoid (SP)	Lateral sphenobasilar (LSB)*	59
Squamosal (SQ)	Temporoparietal, ant. (TPA)*	62
Stylohyoid (SH)	Stylohyoid (SH)	49
Subclavius (SUBC)	Subclavius (SCL)*	107
Subscapularis (SUB)	Subscapularis (SUB)	111
Supraorbital (SO)	Supraorbital (SO)	56
Supraspinatus (SPI)	Supraspinatus medial (SSM)*	119
Talus (TAL)	Talus (TAL)	197
Teres major (TM)	Teres Major (TMA)*	124
Teres minor (TMI)	Teres minor (TMI)	125
Tracheal (TR)	Anterior medial cervical (AMC)*	74
TS3	Infraspinatus inferior (ISI)*	123
Upper pole fifth lumbar (UP5L)	Upper posterior fifth lumbar (UPL5)*	164
Wrist (WRI)	Palmar wrist (PWR)*	136
Zygoma (Z)	Posterior temporalis (PT)*	61

---

*Change in terminology.

¶APPLICATION OF STRAIN AND COUNTERSTRAIN (OR POSITIONAL RELEASE THERAPY) TO THE NEUROLOGIC PATIENT

Adapted from Sharon Weiselfish, Ph.D., P.T.

I COMMON STRAIN AND COUNTERSTRAIN OR PRT TECHNIQUES FOR THE NEUROLOGIC PATIENT

Upper Quadrant

The muscles of the upper quadrant, which, when treated with strain and counterstrain techniques, (or PRT) most efficiently affect spasticity, are as follows:

SCS Terminology	PRT Terminology	Page
Anterior cervicals	AC	65-74
Lateral cervicals (scalenes)	LC	75, 76
Anterior first thoracic	AT1	86
Elevated first rib	PR1	101
Second depressed rib	AR2	92
Pectoralis minor	PMI	116
Subscapularis	SUB	111
Latissimus dorsi (subluxed hemiplegic shoulder)	LD	117
Third depressed rib	AR3	93
Biceps	BLH, BSH	110, 114

Lower Quadrant

The muscles of the lower quadrant, which, when treated with strain and counterstrain techniques, (or PRT) most efficiently affect spasticity, are as follows:

SCS Terminology	PRT Terminology	Page
Sacral tender points	PS1-PS5 COX	175-180
Quadratus lumborum	QL	161
Iliacus	IL	151
Piriformis	PRM, PRL	171
Adductor	ADD	158
Medial hamstrings	MH	187
Quadriceps	PAT	183
Gastrocnemius (extended ankle)	PAN	198
Medial ankle	MAN	194
Flexed calcaneus	PCA	207
Medial calcaneus	MCA	205
Talus	TAL	197

II Pathokinesiologic Model

EXAMPLES

1. If the patient has a protracted shoulder girdle and there is a limitation in horizontal abduction, it is assumed that the pectoralis minor is hypertonic with shortened and contracted muscle fibers. The technique of a second depressed rib would be utilized to decrease the gamma gain of the pectoralis minor. AR2 Page 92

2. If the patient has an anteriorly displaced humeral head with an internally rotated shoulder joint and limitation in external rotation, the technique for subscapularis would be utilized. SUB Page 111

3. If the patient has a limitation in shoulder abduction and a depressed humeral head or a caudal subluxation/dislocation of the glenohumeral joint, the techniques for the latissimus dorsi and the third depressed rib would be utilized. LD Page 117, AR3 Page 93

4. If the patient has an elevated shoulder girdle and there is a limitation in cervical side bending to the opposite side, the lateral cervical techniques would be utilized, to decrease the gamma gain for the medial scalenes, which elevate the first rib. LC2-6 Page 76

5. If the proximal head of the first rib is elevated, rib excursion with respiration is inhibited, and lower cervical range of motion—especially rotation—is limited, the technique for an elevated first rib (PR1) can be utilized. PR1 Page 101

6. If the patient has a flexed elbow joint and a limitation in elbow extension, the technique for the biceps can be utilized. BLH Page 110, BSH Page 114

7. If the patient has a pronated forearm and a limitation of forearm supination, the points for the medial epicondyle can be utilized. Often the proximal radial head is displaced anterior, as a compensatory movement. The technique for the radial head (RHS, RHP) can be utilized. RHS Page 129, RHP Page 130

8. If the patient has an elevated pelvic girdle with a limitation of lumbar side bending to the opposite side, the technique for the quadratus lumborum (the anterior twelfth thoracic tender point) can be utilized. AT12 Page 89

9. If the patient has a hip flexion tightness or contracture with a limitation of hip extension, the technique for the iliacus can be utilized. IL Page 151

10. If the patient has an adducted and internally rotated hip and there is a limitation of external rotation of the hip, the technique for the adductor can be utilized. ADD Page 158

11. If the patient has a flexion synergic pattern of spasticity at the knee and there is a limitation of knee extension, the point for the medial hamstrings can be utilized. MH Page 187

12. If the patient has an extensor synergic pattern of spasticity at the knee with a limitation of flexion, the technique for the quadriceps (patella extensors) can be utilized. PAT Page 183

13. If the patient has an equinus posture with a plantar flexed foot and a limitation in dorsiflexion, the technique for the medial gastrocnemius (PAN) can be utilized. PAN Page 198

14. If the patient has an equinovarus foot posture with a limitation in eversion, the technique for the medial ankle and medial calcaneus can be utilized. MAN Page 194, MCA Page 205

15. If the patient has a clubfoot with an internal rotated and dropped talus, the technique for the talus can be utilized. TAL Page 197

¶THE IMPORTANCE OF SOFT TISSUES FOR STRUCTURAL SUPPORT OF THE BODY

Stephen M. Levin, M.D.

From the Potomac Back
Center
Vienna, Virginia

Reprint requests to:
Stephen M. Levin, M.D.
Director
Potomac Back Center
1577 Springhill Road
Vienna, VA 22182

Most of us view the skeleton as the frame upon which the soft tissues are draped. The post-and-beam construction of a skyscraper is the favored model for the spine[11] and is used for all biologic structures—the upright spine is regarded as the highest biomechanical achievement. The soft tissues are regarded as stabilizing "guy wires," similar to the curtain walls of steel-framed buildings (Fig. 1).

Skyscrapers are immobile, rigidly hinged, high-energy–consuming, vertically oriented structures that depend on gravity to hold them together. The mechanical properties are Newtonian, Hookian, and linear.[4,5] A skyscraper's flagpole or any weight that cantilevers off the building creates a bending moment in the column that produces instability. The building must be rigid to withstand even the weight of a flag blowing in the wind. The heavier or farther out the cantilever, the stronger and more rigid the column must be (Fig. 2). A rigid column requires a heavy base to support the incumbent load. The weight of the structure produces internal shear forces that are destabilizing and require energy just to keep the structure intact (Fig. 3).

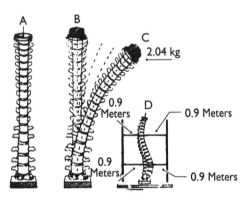

FIG. 1 (Left). *Adult thoracolumbar ligamentous spine, fixed at the base and free at top, under vertical loading, and restrained at midthoracic and midlumbar levels in the anteroposterior plane.* **A,** *before loading.* **B,** *during loading.* **C,** *stability failure occuring under a load of 2.04 kg.* **D,** *lateral view showing anteroposterior restraints.* (From Morris JM, Markolk KL: Biomechanics of the lumbar spine. In American Academy of Orthopaedic Surgeons: Atlas of Orthotics: Biomechanical Principles and Application. St. Louis, Mosby, 1975: with permission.)

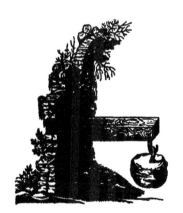

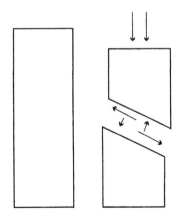

FIG. 2 (Above, left). *Bending stresses in a beam.* (From Galileo: Discorci e dimonstrazioni matematiche intorno a due nuove scienze. Leiden, 1638.)

FIG. 3 (Above, right). *When simple compressive load is applied, both compressive and shear stresses must exist on planes that are oriented obliquely to the line of application to the load.*

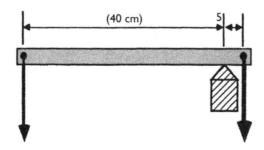

FIG. 4. *A log of 200 kg located 40 cm from the fulcrum requires a muscle reaction force of 8 x 200 = kg. The erectores spinae group can generate a force of about 200-400 kg, which is only a quarter to half of the force that is necessary. Therefore, muscle power alone cannot lift such a load, and another supporting member is required.* (Courtesy of Serge Gracovetsky, PhD.)

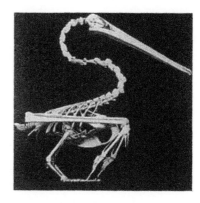

FIG. 5. *Bird Skeleton.* (Courtesy of California Academy of Sciences, San Francisco.)

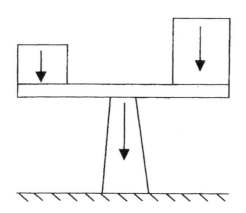

FIG. 6. *Balancing compressive loads.*

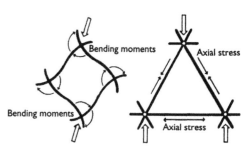

FIG. 7. *Loading a square and a triangular (truss) frame.*

Biologic structures are mobile, flexibly hinged, low-energy–consuming, omnidirectional structures that can function in a gravity-free environment. The mechanical properties are non-Newtonian, non-Hookian, and nonlinear.[5] If a human skeletal system functions as a lever, reaching out a hand or casting a fly at the end of a rod is impossible. The calculated forces with such acts break bone, rip muscle, and deplete energy (Fig. 4). A post-and-beam cannot be used to model the neck of a flamingo, the tail of a monkey, the wing of a bat, or the spine of a snake (Fig. 5). Because invertebrates do not have bones, there is no satisfactory model to adequately explain the structural intergrity of a worm. Post-and-beam modeling in biologic structures could only apply in a perfectly balanced, rigidly hinged, upright spine (Fig. 6). Mobility is out of the equation. The forces needed to keep a column whose center of gravity is constantly changing and whose base is rapidly moving horizontally are overwhelming to contemplate. If we add that the column is composed of many rigid bodies that are hinged together by flexible, almost frictionless joints, the forces are incalculable.[2] The complex cantilevered beams of horizontal spines of quadrupeds and cervical spines in any vertebrate require tall, rigid masts for support[2] that are not usually available.

Since post-and-beam construction has limited use in biologic modeling, other structural models must be explored to determine if a more widely applicable construct can be found. Thompson[14] and, later, Gordon[4] use a truss system similar to those used in bridges for modeling the quadruped spine. Trusses have clear advantages over the post-and-lintel construction of skyscrapers as a structural support system for biologic tissue. Trusses have flexible, even frictionless hinges with no bending moments about the joint. The support elements are either in tension or compression only. Loads applied at any point are distributed about the truss as tension or compression (Fig. 7). In post-and-beam construction, the load is locally loaded and

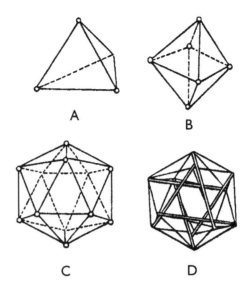

FIG. 8.   A, *tetrahedron,* **B,** *octahedron,* **C,** *icosahedron,* and **D,** *tension-vectored icosahedron with compression elements within the tension shell.*

creates leverage. There are no levers in a truss, and the load is distributed throughout the structure. A truss is fully triangulated, inherently stable, and cannot be bent without producing large deformations of individual members. Since only trusses are inherently stable with freely moving hinges, it follows that any stable structure with freely moving hinges must be a truss. Vertebrates with flexible joints must therefore be constructed as trusses.

When the tension elements of a truss are wires or ropes, the truss usually becomes unidiredtional (see Fig. 7); the element that is under tension will be under compression when turned topsy-turvy. The tension elements of the body (the soft tissues—fascia, muscles, ligaments, and connective tissue) have largely been ignored as construction members of the body frame and have been viewed only as the motors. In loading a truss the elements that are in tension can be replaced by flexible materials such as ropes, wires, or in biologic systems, ligaments, muscles, and fascia. Therefore, the tension elements are an integral part of the construction and not just a secondary support. However, ropes and soft tissue can only function as tension elements, and most trusses constructed with tension members will only function when oriented in one direction. They could not function as mobile, omnidirectional structures necessary for biologic functions. There is a class of trusses called *tensegrity*[3] structures that are omnidirectional so that the tension elements always function in tension regardless of the direction of applied force. A wire bicycle wheel is a familiar example of a tensegrity structure. The compression elements in tensegrity structures "float" in a tension network just as the hub of a wire wheel is suspended in a tension network of spokes.

To conceive of an evolutionary system construction of tensegrity trusses that can be used to model biologic organisms, we must find a tensegrity truss that can be linked in a hierarchical construction. It must start at the smallest subcellular component and must have the potential, like the beehive, to build itself. The structure would be an integrated tensegrity truss that evolved from infinitely smaller trusses that could be, like the beehive cell, both structurally independent and interdependent at the same time. This repetion of forms, like in a hologram, helps in visualizing the evolutionary progression of complex forms from simple ones. This holographic concept seems to apply to the truss model as well.

Architect Buckminster Fuller[3] and sculptor Kenneth Snelson[13] described the truss that fits these requirements, the tensegrity icosahedron. In this structure, the outer shell is under tension, and the vertices are held apart by internal compression "struts" that seem to float in the tension network (Fig. 8).

The tensegrity icosahedron is a naturally occurring, fully triangulated, three-dimensional truss. It is an omnidirectional, gravity-independent, flexibly hinged structure whose mechanical behavior is nonlinear, non-Newtonian, and non-Hookian. Independently, Fuller and

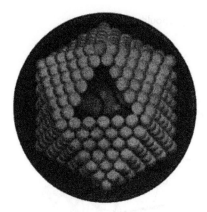

FIG. 9. *The icosahedral structure of a virus.*

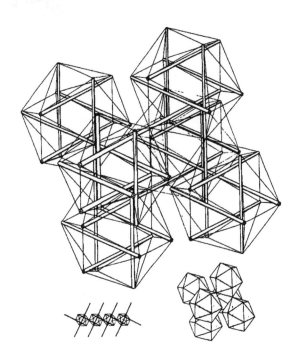

FIG. 10. *Indefinitely extensive array of tensegrity icosahedra.* (From Fuller RB: Synergetics. New York, Macmillan, 1975; with permission.)

Snelson use this truss to build complex structures. Fuller's familiar geodesic dome is an example, and Snelson [12] has used it for artistic sculptures that can be seen around the world. Ingber[7,16] and colleagues use the icosahedron for modeling cell construction. Research is underway to use this structure in more complex tissue modeling.[16] Naturally occurring examples that have already been recognized as icosahedra are the self-generating fullerenes (carbon$_{60}$ organic molecules),[8] viruses,[17] clethrins,[1] cells,[15] radiolaria,[6] pollen grains, dandelion balls, blowfish, and several other biologic structures[9] (Fig. 9).

Icosahedra are stable even with frictionless hinges and, at the same time, can easily be altered in shape or stiffness merely by shortening or lengthening one or several tension elements. Icosahedra can be linked in an infinite variety of sizes or shapes in a modular or hierarchical pattern with the tension elements (the muscles, ligaments, and fascia) forming a continuous interconnecting network and with the compression elements (the bones) suspended within that network (Fig. 10). The structure would always maintain the characteristics of a single icosahedron. A shaft, such as a spine, may be built that is omnidirectional and can function equally well in tension or compression with the internal stresses always distributed in tension or compression. Because there are no bending moments within a tensegrity structure, they have the lowest energy costs.

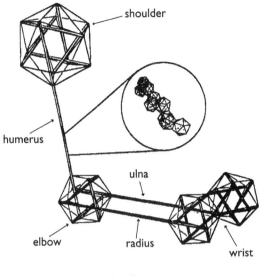

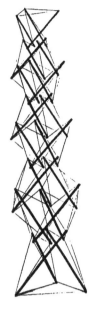

Fig. 11. *Icosa arm.*

FIG. 12. *E-C column.* (Courtesy of Kenneth Snelson.)

Viewed as a model for the spine of humans or any vertebrate species, the tension icosahedron space truss (Fig. 11) with the bones acting as the compressive elements and the soft tissues as the tension elements will be stable in any position, even with multiple joints. They can be vertical or horizontal and assume any posture from ramrod straight to a sigmoid curve (Fig. 12). Shortening one soft tissue element has a rippling effect throughout the structure. Movement is created and a new, instantly stable shape is achieved. It is highly mobile, omnidirectional, and consumes low energy. Tension icosahedrons are unique structures whose constructs, when used as a biologic model, would conform to the natural laws of least energy, laws of mechanics, and the distinct characteristics of biologic tissues. The icosahedron space truss is present in biologic structures at the cellular, subcellular, and multicellular levels. Recent research on the molecular structures of organisms such as viruses, subcellular organelles, and whole organisms has shown them to be icosahedra. The very building block of bone, hydroxyapatite, is an icosahedron. In the spine, each subsystem (vertebrae, disks, soft tissues) would be subsystems of the spine metasystem. Each would function as an icosahedron independently and as part of the larger system, as in the beehive analogy.

The icosahedron space truss spine model is a universal, modular, hierarchical system that has the widest application with the least energy cost. As the simplest and least energy-consuming system, it becomes the metasystem to which all other systems and subsystems must be judged and, if they are not simpler, more adaptable, and less energy consuming, rejected. Since this system always works with the least energy requirements, there would be no benefit to nature for spines to function sometimes as a post, sometimes as a beam, sometimes as a truss, or to function differently for different species, conforming to the minimal inventory-maximum diversity concept of Pearce[10] and evolutionary theory.

The icosahedron space truss model could be extended to incorporate other anatomic and physiologic systems. For example, as a "pump" the icosahedron functions remarkably like cardiac and respiratory models, and, so, may be an even more fundamental metasystem for biologic modeling. As suggested by Kroto,[8] the icosahedron template is "mysterious, ubiquitous, and all powerful."

References

1. de Duve C: A Guided Tour of the Living Cell. Vol. 1. New York, Scientific Books, 1984.
2. Fielding WJ, Burstein AH, Frankel VH: The nuchal ligament. Spine 1:3-14, 1976.
3. Fuller, RB: Synergetics. New York, Macmillan, 1975.
4. Gordon, JE: Structures or Why Things Don't Fall Down. New York, De Capa Press, 1978.
5. Gordon, JE: The Science of Structures and Materials. New York, Scientific American Library, 1988.
6. Haeckel E: Report on the scientific results of the voyage of the H.M.S. Challenger. Vol 18, pt XL. Radiolaria, Edinburgh, 1887.
7. Ingber DE, Jamieson J: Cells as tensegrity structures. Architectural regulation of histodifferentiation by physical forces transduced over basement membrane. In Andersonn LL, Gahmberg CG, Kblom PE (eds): Gene Expression During Normal and Malignant Differentiation. New York, Academic Press, 1985, pp 13-30.
8. Kroto H: Space, stars, C_{60}, and soot. Science 242:1139-1145, 1988.
9. Levin SM: The icosahedron as the three-dimensional finite element in bio-mechanical support. Proceedings of the Society of General Systems Research Symposium on Mental Images, Values and Reality, Philadelphia, 1986. St. Louis, Society of General Systems Research, 1986, pp G14-G26.
10. Pearce PL: Structure in Nature as a Strategy for Design. Cambridge, MA, MIT Press, 1978.
11. Schultz AB: Biomechanics of the spine. In Nelson L (ed): Low Back Pain and Industrial and Social Disablement. London, American Back Pain Association, 1983, pp 20-25.
12. Schultz DG, Fox HN: Kenneth Snelson, Albright-Knox Art Gallery (catalogue), Buffalo, 1981.
13. Snelson KD: Continuous tension, discontinuous compression structures. U.S. Patent 3,169,611, Washington, DC, U.S. Patent Office, 1965.
14. Thompson D: On Growth and Form. Cambridge, Cambridge University Press, 1961.
15. Wang N, Butler JP, Ingber DE: Microtransduction across the cell surface and through the cytoskeleton. Science 260:1124-1127, 1993.
16. Wendling S: Personal communication. Laboratory of Physical Mechanics, Faculty of Science and Technology, Paris.
17. Wildy P, Home RW: Structure of animal virus particles. Prog Med Virol 5:1-42, 1963.

¶OSTEOPATHIC POSITIONING TABLE

Designed by Dr. George Roth and built by Hill Laboratories Co.

This table was specifically designed to reduce practitioner strain and facilitate the practice of PRT. It is available through Hill Laboratories* in Frazer Pennsylvania. A few of the features and possible applications are listed below.

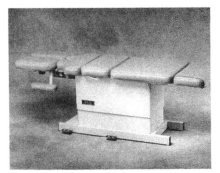

- Multi-sectional
- Motorized elevation 22" to 35"

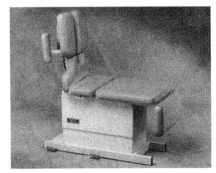

- Motorized thoracic elevation to 85°

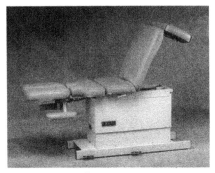

- Leg section flexes to 75°

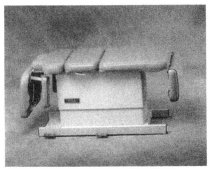

- Head piece adjustable through 135°

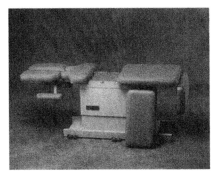

- Removeable pelvic section

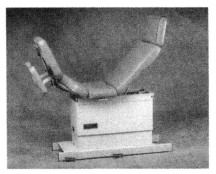

- Wide range of possible positions

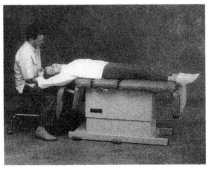

- Anterior/posterior cervical

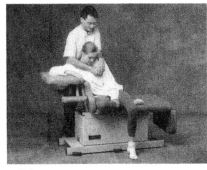

- Rib treatment

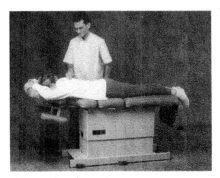

- Posterior thoracic

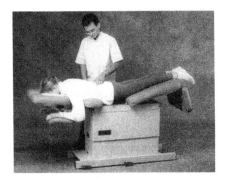

- Posterior lumbar

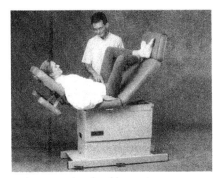

- Anterior lumbar/thoracic

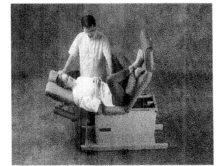

- Iliacus

*Hill Laboratories Co., 3 Bacton Hill Rd., Frazer, Penn., 19355, (610) 644-2867.

Glossary

active myofascial trigger point: A focus of hyperirritability in a muscle or its fascia. An active trigger point is always tender, prevents full lengthening of the muscle, weakens the muscle, usually refers pain on direct compression, mediates a local response of muscle fibers when adequately stimulated, and often produces specific referred autonomic phenomena, generally in its pain reference zone.

acute somatic dysfunction: Immediate or short-term impairment or altered function of related components of the somatic (body framework) system. Characterized in early stages by vasodilation, edema, tenderness, pain, and contraction.

adaptation: The process of attaining homeostasis with respect to changing internal or external circumstances. Adaptation uses the capability of the organism to operate efficiently under altered conditions.

anatomic barrier: The limit of motion imposed by anatomic structure.

articular strain: The result of forces acting on a joint beyond its capacity to adapt. Refers to stretching of joint components beyond physiologic limits, causing damage.

barrier (motion barrier): Limit of unimpeded motion.

biomechanics: The application of mechanical laws to living structures. The study and knowledge of biologic function from an application of mechanical principles.

chiropractic: The science of treating human ailments by manipulation and adjustment of the spine and other structures of the human body. The uses of such other mechanical, physiotherapeutic, dietetic, hygienic, and sanitary measure, except drugs and major surgery, as are incident to the care of the human body.

chronic somatic dysfunction: Long-standing impairment or altered function of related components of the somatic (body framework) system. Characterized by tenderness, itching, fibrosis, paresthesias, and contracture.

comfort zone: The optimal position of ease. It is a position where there is no tenderness and the tissues are completely released. Also called a *position of comfort.*

compensation: Counterbalancing or making up for a defect in structure or function in the body. It may employ mechanisms that meet the definition of adaptation, but it more likely implies adjustment at the expense of efficiency and with greater likelihood of fatigue and wear and tear. Both functional and anatomic breakdown are more likely to occur in a compensated situation

counterstrain technique: An indirect technique developed by Lawrence Jones, D.O. The operator moves the patient or part passively away from the motion barrier toward and into the planes of increased motion, always searching for the position of greatest comfort in order to normalize inappropriate proprioreceptive activity.

cranial technique: A descriptor suggested by W. G. Sutherland, D.O., that refers to management and care (therapy) using manipulative skills applied to the craniosacral mechanism. This form of treatment purports to create shifts in circulation and pressure dynamics of the cerebrospinal fluid and change or normalize pathophysiologic reflexes, structure, and body mechanics.

craniosacral therapy: John Upledger developed craniosacral therapy, which integrates both the osseous and membranous (i.e., meningeal) environment of the central nervous system (i.e., brain and spinal cord). The cranial bones are used as handles to influence the meninges and restore flexibility to the dural tube and its related structures.

craniosacral mechanism: A term used by W.G. Sutherland, D.O., to describe the synchronous movement of the sacral base with the cranial base. This synchrony is accomplished by the attachment of the dural tube to the foramen magnum and sacral canal, probably aided by cerebrospinal fluid fluctuation.

direct technique: Engagement of the restrictive barrier carrying the lesioned component toward or through the barrier. Thrust, articulatory, and muscle energy are examples of direct techniques.

dysfunction: A state of continuing, though not necessarily static, impaired function of a part of the body. Usually involves many local and distant anatomic structures (muscle, fascia, ligaments, viscera, vascular components).

facilitated segment: The altered physiologic state of the neural spinal segment such that it has a lowered threshold to stimulation, being hyperirritable to any stimulation and causing abnormal function in parts it normally affects.

facilitation: (1) An increase in afferent stimuli such that the synaptic threshold is more easily reached; thus there is increase in the efficacy of subsequent impulses in that pathway or synapse. The consequence of increased efficacy is that continued stimulation produces hyperactive responses. (2) A clinical concept used by osteopathic physicians to describe neurophysiologic mechanisms that create or are created by somatic dysfunction. Most often used to describe enhancement or reinforcement of neuronal activity caused by increased or abnormal afferent input to a segment or segments. Increased activity is often triggered or enhanced by adrenergic and sympathetic stimulation.

fine-tuning: Small increments in movement adjustments (i.e., flexion, extension, rotation, lateral flexion, compression, or distraction).

flat palpation: Examination by finger pressure that proceeds across the muscle fibers at a right angle to their length while compressing them against a firm underlying structure, such as bone. Used to detect taut bands and trigger points.

flowerspray endings: Muscle spindle sensory end organs.

gamma efferent: Autonomic nervous system fibers carrying signals from the pyramidal centers, causing alterations of sensitivity and length in the action of muscles via special organs called muscle spindles.

golgi endings: Sensory organs found in tendons of muscles. Act as muscle stretch overload protectors via the spinal reflexes.

homeostasis: (1) Maintenance of static or constant conditions in the internal environment. (2) The level of well-being of an individual maintained by internal physiologic harmony. Result of a relatively stable state or equilibrium among the interdependent body functions.

indirect technique: Any manual technique in which the treating force is directed away from the motion restriction. Sutherland, functional, counterstrain, and positional release therapy are examples of indirect techniques.

inhibition, reflex: (1) In osteopathic usage, a term that describes the application of steady pressure to soft tissues to effect relaxation and normalize reflex activity. (2) Effect on antagonist muscles due to reciprocal innervation when the agonist is stimulated.

joint hypermobility: Signifies increased joint movement.

joint hypomobility: Signifies joint stiffness or relative restriction of motion.

jump sign: A general pain response of the patient (wincing, crying out, or withdrawal of a body part) in response to pressure applied on a trigger point.

latent myofascial trigger point: A focus of hyperirritability in muscle or its fascia that is clinically quiescent with respect to spontaneous pain. Painful only when palpated.

manipulation: Therapeutic application of manual force. Also known as a therapeutic movement usually of a small amplitude; accomplished at the end of the available range of motion but within the anatomic range, at a speed over which the client has no control.

mobilization: Therapeutic movement of variable amplitude accomplished within the available range of motion at a speed over which the client has control.

muscle energy technique: A direct technique developed by Dr. Fred Mitchell, Sr., D.O., used to treat joint hypomobility. This technique involves passively positioning the patient using muscle barriers in a precisely controlled position. Once in this position, a gentle isometric contraction in a specific direction against a specific resistance is required. This results in increased mobility of the pelvis, spine, ribs, and peripheral joints.

muscle spindles: The special neuromuscular organs scattered through the mass of muscle fibers that act not only as a feedback sensor to allow spinal reflexes to adjust intentional or higher reflex muscle contraction orders, but also have sensitivity, or "gain control," which allows them to adapt to new load or new intentional signals from higher centers.

myofascial release: A whole body, hands-on approach for the evaluation and treatment of the fascial system. A three-dimensional soft tissue technique that addresses tension in the connective tissue system and can be either direct or indirect.

myotatic reflex arc: Stretch reflex of the muscle.

osteopathy (osteopathic medicine): A system of health care founded by Andrew Taylor Still (1828–1917). Based on the theory that the body is capable of making its own remedies against disease and other toxic conditions when it is in normal structureal relationship and has favorable environmental conditions and adequate nutrition. Uses generally accepted physical, pharmacologic, and surgical methods of diagnosis and therapy; places strong emphasis on the importance of body mechanics and manipulative methods to detect and correct faulty structure and function. Structure governs function; disturbances of structure, in whatever tissue within the body, lead to disturbances of function in that structure, and in turn of the function of the body as a whole. Supports the body's inherent abilities to maintain homeostasis and to establish a protective response to disease or injury.

osteopathic lesion (osteopathic lesion complex): A disturbance in musculoskeletal structure or function, as well as associated disturbances of other biologic mechanisms.

pain analog scale: Scale used to assist patients with determining level of pain (0 = no pain; 10 = extremely painful).

pathologic barrier: A functional limit within the anatomic range of motion, which abnormally diminishes the normal physiologic range. May be associated with somatic dysfunction.

physical (manual) therapy: Usually part of a multidisciplinary approach using a variety of maneuvers and manual techniques in conjunction with conventional physical therapy modalities. Directed at restoring normal function and arthrokinematics of the somatic system.

physiologic barrier: Functional limits within the anatomic range of motion. Soft tissue tension accumulation, which limits the voluntary motion of an articulation. Further motion toward the anatomic barrier can still be induced passively.

physiologic motion: Normal changes in the position of articulating surfaces taking place within a joint or region.

positional release therapy: A passive and indirect technique that places the patient's body, utilizing all three planes of movement, into a position of greatest comfort. While in this position of comfort, there is a reduction and arrest of inappropriate proprioceptive activity and a release of fascial tension. This results in decreased hypertonicity, relaxation, and elongation of involved muscle fibers. Decreases myofascial tension and helps restore joint mobility. The result is increased functional mobility and flexibility and decreased pain.

position of comfort: The optimal position of ease. A position where there is no tenderness and the tissues are completely released. Also called the comfort zone.

proprioception: The sensing of motion and where the body is positioned in space.

proprioceptor: Sensory nerve terminals that give information concerning movements and position of the body or posture. They occur chiefly in the muscles, tendons, joints, and the labyrinth and provide information with regard to changes in equilibrium and the knowledge of position, weight, and resistance of objects in relation to the body.

protective muscle spasm guarding: The muscle is in a state of contraction, incapable of allowing full resting length due to an inability to relax and elongate. Muscle will resist passive elongation or stretch.

reality check: A positional movement or specific joint, fascial, or muscle evaluation or a pain scale that is objective and can be measured. It reproduces the patient's pain or complaint. Used as a reference point to measure the success of treatment.

reciprocal innervation: The inhibition of antagonist muscles when the agonist is stimulated.

referred pain: Pain that is perceived at some distance from the location of the cause.

release phenomena: A normalization or softening of the tissue. During this process the patient may experience some or all of the following: pain, paresthesia, pulsations, vibrations, heat, perspiration, change in breathing or heart rate, and eye motor activity.

restriction: A resistance or impediment to movement.

segment: A portion of a larger body or structure set off by natural or arbitrarily established boundaries. Often equated with spinal segment. (1) A portion of the spinal cord contained between two imaginary sections, one on each side of a nerve pair. (2) A portion of the spinal cord to which a pair of spinal nerves is attached by dorsal and ventral roots. Also used to describe a single vertebra, namely, a vertebral segment.

somatic dysfunction: Impaired or altered function of related components of the somatic (body framework) system: skeletal, arthrodial, and myofascial structures and related vascular, lymphatic, and neural elements. The positional and motion aspects of somatic dysfunction may be described using three parameters: the position of the element as determined by palpation, the direction in which motion is freer, and the direction in which motion is restricted.

spasm: An involuntary sudden movement or convulsive muscle contraction. Spasms may be clonic (characterized by alternate contraction and relaxation) or tonic (sustained).

spasticity: Increased tone or contractions of muscles causing stiff and awkward movement. The result of an upper motor neuron lesion.

spindle afferent (fibers): Pick up information from the muscle spindle through annulospiral endings and flower-spray endings about the length and contraction of the spindle (and therefore the skeletal muscle fibers), which allows spinal reflex adjustment of muscle tasks desired by higher intentional or reflex centers in the brain.

strain: An overexertion trauma to a portion of the contractile musculotendinous unit or its attachment to the bone (tendinoperiosteal junction). Force that deforms a body part or changes its dimension.

stress: Any force that tends to distort a body. It may be in the direction of either pulling apart or pressing together. Thus skeletal structures (bones, ligaments, and muscles) may be subject to stress or may transmit a stress.

stretching: Separation of the origin and insertion of a muscle or attachment of fascia or ligaments by applying constant pressure at a right angle to the fibers of the muscle or fascia.

tender point: A tender edematous region located deep in muscle, tendons, ligaments, fascia, and bone. It can measure 1 cm across or less, with most acute points being about 3 mm in diameter.

trigger point (myofascial trigger point): A small hypersensitive site that when stimulated consistently produces a reflex mechanism that gives rise to referred pain or other manifestations. The response is specific, in a constant reference zone, and consistent from person to person.

visceral manipulation: A soft tissue technique developed by Jean Pierre Barral, D.O. Involves locating and treating areas of fascial tension in the chest, abdomen, and pelvic cavities to improve functional mobility and visceral function.

Index

Printed and bound by CPI Group (UK) Ltd, Croydon, CR0 4YY

03/10/2024

01040354-0020